IT'S UP TO YOU

Overcoming
Erection Problems

IT'S UP TO YOU

**Overcoming
Erection Problems**

WARWICK WILLIAMS
B.Sc. (Med) M.B. B.S. D.A. F.R.A.N.Z.C.P.
Consultant Psychiatrist and Sex Therapist, Sydney

THORSONS PUBLISHING GROUP

First published in the United Kingdon 1989

Original Australian edition published by Williams & Wilkins,
Adis Pty Limited, 404 Sydney Road, Balgowlah, NSW 2093, Australia.

British Library Cataloguing in Publication Data

Williams, Warwick
    It's up to you.
    1. Men. Impotence. Self treatment
    I. Title
    616.6'9

ISBN 0 7225 1915 X

Published by Thorsons Publishers Limited, Wellingborough,
Northamptonshire, NN8 2RQ, England

Printed in Great Britain by Billing & Sons Limited, Worcester

10 9 8 7 6 5 4 3 2 1

Editorial Preface

Men who suffer erection problems often feel isolated and dejected, but such problems are very much more common than most people realise. Across all ages, probably as many as one in ten men suffer erection problems. At one time these problems were considered to be almost entirely psychological but we now know that many cases result from physical causes. It is encouraging that in recent years major advances have been made in understanding how erection occurs and how to treat erection problems so that now the majority of sufferers can be helped.

Many men can overcome their erection problems by self-help programmes. *It's up to You* is the best self-help book especially written for men with erection problems I have come across. The author, an experienced sex therapist and doctor, gives detailed advice and a step-by-step series of exercises which, followed carefully, should help men to regain enjoyable sexual activity.

I do not hesitate to commend this book not only to men suffering erection problems, and their partners, but also to those professionals who are involved in helping them. The adage that prevention is better than cure applies to sexual issues. Followed carefully, the guidance given by Dr Warwick Williams will help the reader continue satisfying sexual activity way into old age.

Dr Alan J Riley
Specialist in Sexual Medicine
Editor, British Journal of Sexual Medicine
and joint editor, Sexual and Marital Therapy

Foreword

'If you can't get it up when you want and keep it up for as long as you want, you're just a hopeless failure.' This quotation is typical of statements made by many men who seek help for impotence. Problems with a man's erection can cause profound psychological disturbance, particularly in our society. Many men believe that if they fail to obtain an erection 'on demand' they are no longer real men. They see a dark future of dismal failure and subdued, or open, derision by their friends, should they learn about their disability. Some men who have erection failure believe that this will induce their partner to seek sexual consolation with other men. Many become depressed.

Although it is now known that about half of all men who have problems with erection have as significant contributory causes a medical illness, heavy smoking or drinking, or prescribed medications, in the remaining cases, psychological problems are mainly responsible. Effective treatment must address all relevant issues.

Warwick Williams has had a vast experience in identifying and overcoming the causes of men's erection problems. Aware of the destructive nature of impotency, he has written this book so that men can help themselves.

Sexual problems can be resolved if, first, the afflicted person seeks professional guidance; second, if he takes heed of the advice given; and third, if he follows an appropriate programme of exercises. In this book the author gives detailed guidance and advice, plus a step-by-step series of exercises, which, if followed, have a high chance of restoring a man's potency, to his and to his partner's joy.

This is a superb book: clearly written and splendidly direct, it will help many men overcome their erection problems. However, it must be read with care and the instructions followed in the manner the author suggests.

DEREK LLEWELLYN-JONES

Contents

Introduction

The material in this book is the result of many years experience in working with men troubled by erection problems.

It is directed primarily at afflicted men, and their partners, if any, aiming to give them real hope, a working understanding of the problem, and most importantly, step-by-step detailed instructions for overcoming the difficulty.

I hope that those in the various helping professions will also find the treatment approaches suggested useful, since there is little available giving explicit, detailed therapeutic instructions and providing a programmed, sequential treatment approach.

I would like to thank all those who have helped and inspired me, particularly Dr John Ellard for suggesting that the book be written and encouraging me to do it, Dr Derek Richardson for constructively reviewing the manuscript, Professor Derek Llewellyn-Jones for writing the foreword, Pamela Petty from Williams & Wilkins, ADIS for invaluable editorial advice and assistance, Penny Zylstra for doing the illustrations, and last, but certainly not least, my wife Elizabeth, who made many suggestions, did all the typing, and uncomplainingly made available the time needed to convert my ideas and experience into print. Of course, everything really important that I know has ultimately been learned from my patients, to whom I am deeply indebted.

WARWICK WILLIAMS
May, 1985

Chapter 1

WHY SELF-HELP?

Erection problems occur very commonly, increasingly so as men get older. The effects of persistent impotence can be devastating and far reaching, often adversely affecting self-confidence, marital happiness, mental health and even such things as performance at work. It is a problem which in many ways hits at men in the area in which they are most vulnerable.

There is little of worth written on impotence in the popular press, and men are much less frequently exposed than are women to accurate information on their sexual problems. This unhappy situation is compounded by the fact that myths and misleading information on impotence and related issues abound and are widespread in the community.

From the medical point of view, impotence is often an exceedingly complex problem, and is becoming more so with the advance of knowledge. Medical courses do not equip future medical practitioners to deal adequately with the problem, giving them only a basic idea of the issues involved and the broad principles of treatment.

Even if the impotent man can overcome his anxiety and embarrassment to a degree sufficient to enable him to discuss the problem with his family doctor, many such physicians have not had the necessary postgraduate training to enable them to handle the problem proficiently. This often leads to referral to one of a variety of specialists, but problems do not then cease, since no single medical specialty possesses all the necessary diagnostic and treatment skills required. Many specialists have had no formal training in the management of these problems, and often all they can do is exclude or deal with relevant abnormalities in their own narrow field of expertise. There are but few trained therapists specializing in the treatment of sexual problems, making the task of getting their help difficult because of long waiting lists.

In spite of all this, the fact remains that many cases of impotence can be overcome using relatively simple treatment techniques. Modern sex therapy relies heavily on the prescription and performance of homework exercises, and the bulk of the treatment is actually done at home by the person himself, under guidance. If an impotent male has a detailed step-by-step description of what he must do to overcome his problem, then the need for consultations with a trained therapist can in many cases be overcome or greatly reduced.

It cannot be emphasized too strongly that a **great deal** can often be achieved using self-help procedures, **provided** they are fully understood, and **performed absolutely correctly!** Over many years of clinical practice, I have developed a tremendous respect for a person's ability to help himself and resolve his problems using his own personal resources. All that a therapist contributes sometimes is a little guidance. In keeping with this experience, the aim of this book is to make readily available a wide range of self-help techniques so that men with erection problems can help themselves, almost as if they were being personally guided by an experienced therapist. There are, of course, situations in which medical investigation and treatment, and specialized assistance are required, and these will be clearly indicated.

While this book is essentially directed at heterosexual males, the issues, principles and techniques are equally relevant for, and applicable to, homosexual men.

Chapter 2

HOW TO GET THE MAXIMUM POSSIBLE BENEFIT FROM THIS BOOK

Lengthy experience in working with many impotent patients has taught me that the best results are achieved by following certain guidelines or principles.

Could I suggest that you will get the maximum benefit if you adhere as closely as possible to the suggestions which follow.

1. Start at the very beginning. Do not skip any chapters! You **must** understand the relevant issues **before** you can be helped by the do-it-yourself exercises. The early sections cover briefly the minimum basic knowledge you simply must have if you are to be assisted by the exercises, so resist the temptation simply to skim through them. The book is so arranged, that to get the full benefit from any chapter, you **must** have read, **and thoroughly understood, all** the chapters before it.

2. When in a chapter you come to an exercise, do it before you read any further! **Do not** bypass the exercises and try to read the whole book first! The exercises are **absolutely essential** for success and you will get very little indeed from merely reading the text.

3. Make haste slowly! Do not rush through the book and the exercises. Remember, you are playing for high stakes — your future sexual happiness! No matter how much spare time you

have to read and practise the exercises, you must realize that it will probably take at least several months to regain your confidence in your sexual ability and improve your potency.

4. Do the exercises **exactly** as instructed. Resist the temptation to do them your own way! They are based on a great deal of experience working with men over many years, and there are important reasons for them being done the way they are described.

5. If you have a partner, discuss with her, on a chapter-by-chapter basis, those issues which apply to you.

6. Do the exercises under good conditions! Do **not** attempt them if you are tired, preoccupied with problems, or feeling upset or unwell. To get the maximum benefit you must be able to concentrate and apply all your resources to what you are doing.

7. The best way to read the book and perform the exercises, is to **do a little frequently** — perhaps half to one hour most days. This is **far more effective** than infrequent but lengthy periods of reading or doing the exercises.

8. In a notebook, keep a detailed written record of what you actually do from this book, on a day-to-day basis. This will act as a constant reminder of what has to be done, and of your progress.

Good luck!

Chapter 3

WHAT YOU NEED TO KNOW ABOUT THE STRUCTURE AND FUNCTIONING OF THE PENIS

Before you can properly understand what can go wrong to produce impotence, you must have a basic knowledge of the construction and operation of the penis. Basically it consists of 3 cylinders bound together by an outer sheath, and covered by skin. One cylinder lies on the under-surface of the penis and surrounds the urinary passage or urethra. The other 2 cylinders lie on the sides and upper surface of the penis, side by side. They are essentially pressure chambers which become inflated with blood when the penis erects. These structures are shown diagrammatically in figure 1.

The cylinder containing the urinary passage is very slender as it passes through the visible part of the penis, but it expands considerably at the end of the penis to form the head or glans. It is also greatly enlarged at its other end, located out of sight underneath the bones of the pelvis, forming what is known as the bulb of the penis. Figure 2 shows its shape.

The pressure cylinders concerned with erection lie side by side in the visible part of the penis, but underneath the pelvis they separate to attach to the pelvic bones — see figures 3 and 4.

Underneath the pelvis, covering those parts of the three penile cylinders lying separately there, are several very important muscles, lying beneath the bases of the cylinders. These muscles have

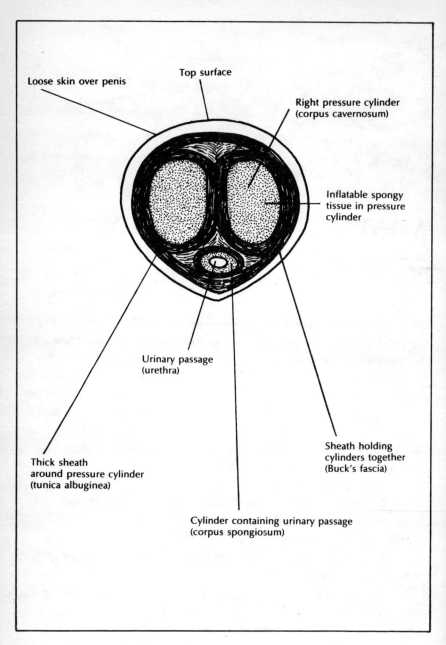

Fig. 1 Diagrammatic cross-section of the penis

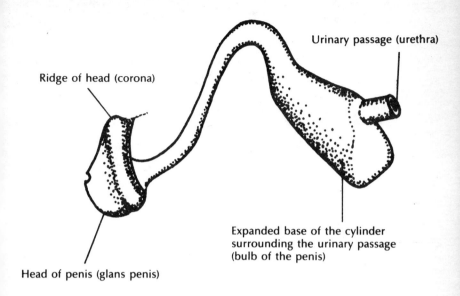

Urinary passage (urethra)

Ridge of head (corona)

Expanded base of the cylinder
surrounding the urinary passage
(bulb of the penis)

Head of penis (glans penis)

*Fig. 2 Side view of the penile cylinder surrounding the urinary
passage (corpus spongiosum)*

complex technical names, (bulbospongiosus, ischiocavernosus) but
may simply be called the major penile muscles. They have important
functions in ejaculation and probably also in the process of erection.

Towards the tip of the penis, the blunt ends of the two pressure
cylinders fit under the expanded end or glans of the penis, which
fits like a cap over them.

The penis contains many blood vessels and nerves. The nerves
are of two broad types. Some control the penile blood vessels,
regulating blood flow through the penis. Others are activated when
the penis is stimulated, sending messages about touch, warmth,
pressure and so on back to the spinal cord and brain.

The blood vessels of the penis are in essence tubes of variable
size, which take fresh blood from the heart to the penis (penile
arteries), and used blood back to the heart (penile veins).

Unless a man has been circumcised, the glans or head of the penis
is covered to some degree by the foreskin or prepuce. In some men

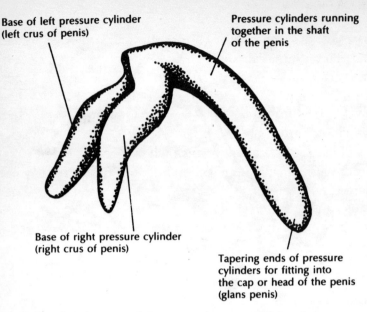

Base of left pressure cylinder
(left crus of penis)

Pressure cylinders running
together in the shaft
of the penis

Base of right pressure cylinder
(right crus of penis)

Tapering ends of pressure
cylinders for fitting into
the cap or head of the penis
(glans penis)

*Fig. 3 Side view of the two pressure cylinders of the penis
(corpora cavernosa)*

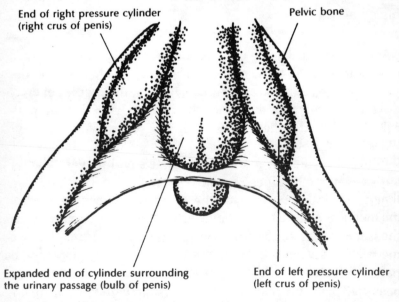

End of right pressure cylinder
(right crus of penis)

Pelvic bone

Expanded end of cylinder surrounding
the urinary passage (bulb of penis)

End of left pressure cylinder
(left crus of penis)

*Fig. 4 Upside-down view of the three penile cylinders at their
bases, underneath the bones of the pelvis*

this is very long, in others quite short, both variations being absolutely normal. The foreskin should be able to be pulled right back over the head of the penis, without any difficulty or discomfort. If it cannot, there may be a problem needing medical attention.

The skin over the shaft of the non-erect penis is very loose, and can easily be moved up and down over the surface of the penis. This is of great practical importance when it comes to learning the correct erotic technique for effectively stimulating a non-erect penis.

There is an enormous variation in the size of the normal penis, both erect and non-erect, just as there is in the height of normal men. Many males worry that their penis is too small, failing to realize that the size of their organ has got nothing to do with its erotic usefulness and their capabilities as a lover! For some men, having a big penis is like having big arm muscles — something mainly of ornamental value, used to boost self-esteem! Self-dissatisfied owners of smaller penises may be surprised to know that during lovemaking a large organ can actually be a real disadvantage, making penetration uncomfortable and intercourse difficult. Women in general are not fussed about size, regarding as much more important the skill and considerateness with which the penis is used, and the emotional aspects of lovemaking.

How Does an Erection Occur from Sexual Stimulation?

There are two basic mechanisms operating. The main one involves messages (or nerve impulses) being transmitted from the brain, down through the spinal cord, and out along nerves running from the spinal cord to the blood vessels of the penis. This results in more blood flowing into the penis than can get out, producing an erection by inflating the 2 pressure cylinders. The third cylinder, and therefore the glans of the penis, is also expanded to some degree. The second mechanism involves the stimulation of nerves in the penis and other parts of the genital area, resulting in nerve messages or impulses being fed into the relevant parts of the spinal cord and brain.

The brain is without doubt **the most important** sexual organ in the body, being ultimately responsible for the physical changes associated with sexual arousal and functioning, and for the all-important emotional accompaniments. In addition to connections from the brain to the penis, which when activated lead to erection, there are other connections which block or inhibit the development of an erection, or lead to the loss of an already established erection. These inhibitory connections are exceedingly important, since their activation by such things as anxiety, anger, unhelpful thoughts or off-putting memories, can lead to impotence. This can occur when there is absolutely nothing wrong with the penis and its controlling mechanisms, and in spite of effective sexual stimulation.

During lovemaking the degree of erection normally fluctuates considerably, depending on the intensity of the combined mental and physical stimulation being received at any given moment.

The process of erection is of course much more complex than described, and some aspects of it are poorly understood.

Erections During Sleep

Whether or not we remember them, we all have dreams while we sleep. In or around the phase of sleep where we dream, in the normal male, the penis becomes firmly erect. Just how this occurs is not understood. Sophisticated measurement of the degree of erection achieved during sleep can sometimes provide useful information about the cause of erection problems when a man is awake.

Early Morning Erections

Just why these occur in normal men is incompletely understood. It is popularly assumed that such an erection is due to a full bladder — hence the term 'piss-horn'. The actual mechanisms leading to such early morning erections are probably much more complex. A common misconception is that if an impotent man awakens with a complete erection, then there cannot be anything physically wrong with him contributing to his erection problem. **This is simply not true!** For example, some men whose impotence results from a spinal cord injury, can have normal early morning erections.

The Role of Hormones in Normal Erection

Hormones are essentially chemicals produced in particular body organs, such as the thyroid gland or testicle, which have important effects on other body organs. They are released into the blood, which carries them to where they are needed. The body produces many hormones, and their exact effects (if any) on the erection mechanism are very complex. It is a fact that a variety of hormone abnormalities can lead to impotence in some men, although the mechanism of this effect may be very indirect—for example, in diabetes—or unknown.

The Mechanism of an Erection Going Down ('Detumescence')

In the normal course of events, an erection will go down either when stimulation (mental or physical) ceases, or after orgasm and ejaculation. These effects are brought about by changes in the blood vessels in the penis, these being controlled by the brain and spinal cord, through the nerves to the penis.

After a man has ejaculated, there is normally what is technically called a 'refractory period', during which further erection is impossible, no matter how much he is stimulated and how aroused he becomes. This period may be quite short in young men, but tends to get longer as a man ages — it may eventually last for more than a day in some men.

The Independence of Erection and Ejaculation/Orgasm

Normally, ejaculation (the pumping out of seminal fluid) and the associated pleasurable feelings, orgasm, occur while a man has an erection. However, even without an erection, a man can still ejaculate normally and experience a normal orgasm, **provided** he is adequately sexually stimulated. This is crucially important knowledge for men with erection problems (and their partners), because it means that even without an erection, lovemaking (or masturbation) can proceed to a pleasurable sexual climax with release of sexual tension.

The trick in achieving ejaculation and orgasm without an erection lies in manipulating the penis correctly, which will be discussed in chapter 12.

Exceptions to the rule that impotent men can be appropriately manipulated to ejaculation and orgasm, occur when some chemical, disease or injury simultaneously affects **both** the processes of erection **and** ejaculation.

Chapter 4

WHAT YOU NEED TO KNOW ABOUT THE EFFECTS OF NORMAL AGEING ON THE PROCESS OF GETTING AND MAINTAINING AN ERECTION

In young adulthood, a man can often achieve a complete erection very rapidly, without any physical touching at all. If he can hold off ejaculation, such a man's erection may last for a considerable time, even if he receives no physical stimulation.

As you grow older however, certain fairly predictable changes tend to occur to your erectile function. The age at which these begin to be noticed varies greatly from man to man, but often they are quite obvious by 40, or sooner, and become increasingly important from then on.

Firstly, with increasing age, it usually takes you longer to obtain an adequate erection. Secondly, more stimulation is normally required. Eventually, direct physical manipulation of the penis will always be needed, as an adequate erection will simply no longer result from purely mental stimulation. Thirdly, the degree of hardness or firmness of a full erection will often decrease a little, although normally it will be still perfectly adequate for penetration. Fourthly, with increasing age, your erection will tend to go down on you, unless you are continuously and adequately stimulated. This change may eventually necessitate your partner continuing to stimulate your penis, while you move to get into position for intercourse. When your erection has gone down, even if ejaculation has not occurred, it may be much more difficult to regain it, regardless of the stimulation used. Finally, the so-called refractory period after ejaculation, when further penile erection is impossible, often tends to increase greatly with age.

It is **crucially** important that all men and women understand that the changes described above are **perfectly normal.** You may not particularly like some of these changes, but there is **absolutely nothing you can do to prevent them,** and you **must** work at living comfortably with them! The implications of these changes for lovemaking are obvious enough and each couple needs to make appropriate ongoing alterations to their lovemaking procedures.

It is **always** desirable sexual technique for the **female** to insert the penis into her vagina, at any age. This is firstly because a man cannot see exactly what he is doing, and if he attempts to insert his penis, he may cause his partner discomfort or even pain. Secondly, when because of the changes associated with increasing age, the penis becomes less rigid than previously, penetration may be much less simple. Many men lose their erection while they fumble about trying to penetrate without the assistance of their partner!

Because of the age-related changes to the erectile process, men as they get older must pay increasingly strict attention to making sure that their 'conditions' for being sexually responsive are reasonably met, **before** making love, a subject which will be discussed in great detail in chapter 6.

With increasing age, there is normally a gradual decline in sexual drive or interest, so that many men feel like lovemaking somewhat less frequently. Attempting lovemaking, with an expectation of achieving an adequate erection, when you don't really feel interested in sex, is setting yourself up for an episode of impotence. Make love **only** because you **genuinely feel like it,** not because you think you should, or to prove something!

Declining Male Hormone Levels with Increasing Age

In general, men as they age do not experience a relatively rapid decline in sex hormone levels, as women do around the change of life. However, the amount of male hormone produced by the body often appears to gradually decrease with age, and in some men (but by no means all) this decrease may contribute to erectile problems. The only way of telling whether or not this is a possibility, is to measure the blood level of male hormone. While this sounds simple enough, it can be extremely difficult to interpret the significance of the result of this blood test. Very few elderly men truly require testosterone (male hormone) replacement therapy.

Other Changes

As men grow older, there are often changes to the processes of ejaculation and orgasm. As a very broad generalization, with increasing age it takes longer to ejaculate, which may actually be a blessing for some! Ejaculation often becomes less powerful — the fluid is not pumped out so strongly, and may eventually merely ooze out. The sensation of orgasm frequently tends to be somewhat decreased in intensity. The 'refractory period' between one ejaculation and the time when ejaculation is once again possible, tends to increase **greatly** with age, often being much longer than the refractory period to the next erection.

It is very important to realize that these changes are normal, because if a man begins to worry about them, the anxiety he generates may interfere with his erections.

Growing Older Sexually in Perspective

Despite the changes described, there is **no** physical reason why men should not continue to have a regular and totally satisfying sex-life until advanced old age, unless of course some illness or disease affecting the sexual apparatus should appear. **The most important factor** in maintaining adequate sexual functioning into advanced old age, is **regular expression of one's sexual needs!** In a sense, the more often you do it, the longer it will last. This, of course, does **not** in any way imply that you should ever try to make yourself perform sexually if you really don't feel like it. To do so is both stupid and a recipe for disaster!

Chapter 5

DESTRUCTIVE SEXUAL MYTHS

It is almost impossible for a man to grow up in today's society without acquiring and believing quite a number of totally ridiculous misconceptions, false notions or myths about sex!

How does this happen? Our sexual attitudes are **learned** — they certainly aren't automatic or instinctive! Our sexual learning takes place from **a very early age** in all sorts of ways, direct and **indirect.** Information is picked up from our friends, older boys (who are just as ignorant), from sexual jokes, glossy magazines, movies, our parent's and other people's behaviour, and so on. The early sexual learning we get from our parents is mostly **negative,** usually consisting of a series of 'don'ts'! We have very little opportunity of being exposed to and picking up **truly accurate information** until we are much older, but by then our attitudes to sex and sexual behaviour are rigidly fixed, set in concrete, and like all early-established beliefs, difficult to change!

Exactly the same things could be said of our early learning about what it is to be a man. **'Real men',** as depicted in the movies and elsewhere, are tough, fearless, unemotional, striving, successful, and of course, super-sexual, endowed with large tireless penises, and enormous sexual appetites. Naturally, women find them totally irresistible! We grow up with this absurd picture of masculinity in our minds, and in consequence, are afraid to be gentle, to show our real feelings, to admit we are scared, and so on, because we believe this would be **'unmanly'**!

I don't think it would be an exaggeration to say that **most** men, **if** they could be completely honest with themselves, would admit to feeling somewhat inadequate, both sexually, and as a man, because of the differences between the way they really are and the way they feel they should be! This self-perceived inadequacy causes us **repeatedly and unthinkingly** to try to prove, to ourselves and the world at large, just how masculine we really are! We may use athletic skill, academic or business achievement, boasting, and of course sex, to enhance our image of ourselves as masculine men! It may come as a surprise to you to realize that for some men, much of the time, their sexual behaviour has got **nothing whatever** to do with sexual desire or sexual tension — it is basically a way of proving their masculinity! Perhaps you can see how this has applied to you at various times in the past — I certainly can!

Let us now consider the worst of the numerous destructive sexual myths we have picked up, and been hood-winked into believing.

Myths About the Penis ('Phallic Phallacies')

Myth 1   The Bigger the Better!

Most men, at least until they finally grow up or give up, are dissatisfied with the size of their penis! Few would not be happier to be, as they say, better hung! The hard facts are, that it's how you use your penis that really counts! Size is **totally irrelevant,** as long as it is neither too big, nor too small to penetrate your partner. Women in general are not fussed about size! What counts to them is lovemaking skill, and the emotional aspects of what to them, is literally **making love!**

If you worry about the size of your penis, this will interfere with your sexual enjoyment and performance. There is **absolutely nothing** you can do to make it bigger, so get on with using what you have got, as pleasurably as possible!

Myth 2   You Should be Able to Get a Hard-On Whenever You Want One!

What a load of absolute rubbish! Do you know anybody who could get an erection if they were naked in a shop window, in front of an audience, and being paid handsomely if they could get it up? **You simply can't make yourself get an erection!** You can merely **allow** your penis to respond, or not respond, as it chooses. Your penis won't respond unless what it needs to stand up is provided, just as your car won't start unless the battery is connected. What it needs in order to become erect will vary from time to time, and change considerably with age.

Myth 3   An Erection is Essential for Good Sex!
Nonsense! With or without an erection, lovemaking with a cared-for partner will be fulfilling and satisfying for you both, **provided** you don't wreck things by insisting on being erect. The only use of a hard-on is to enable you to penetrate your partner, although I suppose in an emergency it could double as a coat-hanger, while you are getting dressed! **You certainly don't need an erection to fulfil your partner and bring her to orgasm, or to reach orgasm yourself!**

Macho Myths

Myth 1   A Man Should Not Show His Feelings!
To do so is believed to be emotional, weak, feminine or even worse, because a **'real man'** is supposed to control his emotions! The fact that many men manage to do so is a tribute to human ingenuity, because it is certainly a most **abnormal** state of affairs. This myth possibly causes men more unhappiness than any other single misconception, and certainly has a **very destructive** effect on many marriages.

  Even animals are sensible enough to show their feelings! Are you going to go on allowing the average dog to be smarter than you? Do yourself a favour — be human, be emotional! You might even get to like it!

Myth 2   A Real Man is Always Horny and Ready for Sex!
It sounds ridiculous when you see it written down, and nobody in their right mind would seriously argue in favour of such nonsense. However, large numbers of men **act** as if they believe it! They expect themselves to be constantly on the look-out for sexual opportunities,

act upon them no matter how busy, preoccupied or tired they are, and be able to respond, perform and enjoy. The truth is almost the opposite — even the horniest men around only truly feel like sex a small proportion of their waking life, and most find it difficult to respond pleasurably under unfavourable circumstances. Remember of course, that **many men use sex for completely non-sexual purposes,** and may copulate, not because they feel aroused or sexually interested, but to relieve tension, because they think it is expected of them, to prove their masculinity, and so on.

Age Myths

There are 2 opposing myths about the sexual effects of ageing, which are both widely believed.

Myth 1   As You Get Older, There is Absolutely No Change in Your Sexual Interest, Response or Performance!

Although few men would agree with this when it is spelt out so bluntly, many act as if they believe it! For example, they worry because at age 45 it takes a while to erect, they can't get properly hard without direct penile stimulation, and it goes down on them when their partner stops playing with it. They do not know that these changes are normal, inevitable, and absolutely nothing to worry about, believing that age should make no difference!

Myth 2   As You Get Older You Lose Interest in Sex and Can't Do it Anymore!

I never cease to be surprised how many otherwise intelligent men believe this. The tragic thing is that if you believe it, it tends to happen, such is the power over us of our thoughts and expectations. The facts about ageing have been spelt out in chapter 4.

Myths About Lovemaking ('Erotic Follies')

There are so many, it is hard to know where to start. Try these:

Myth 1   Lovemaking Ability Comes Naturally!

I presume that men choose to believe this because sex is indeed a natural body function. A wise Frenchman once said that making love is like playing a delicate violin skilfully, and requires about as much tuition and practice! I see no reason to disagree with him in any way! Unfortunately, many men's egos just can't cope with the idea that they might need to **learn** to be sensual and erotic!

Myth 2   Sex Must be Spontaneous!
If you believe this, there is no place for premeditated sex, where you might, for example, have got rid of the kids for the day, moved your stereo into the bedroom so you can play romantic music, chilled a bottle of champagne and taken your favourite erotica out of their hiding place, so you can enjoy them together in bed! While there is absolutely nothing wrong with spontaneous, impulsive sex, such as a quickie in your car before you get home from a dinner party, do not close your mind to the extra joys which can result from planned lovemaking. For some reason, many women are just as hung-up about this as men.

Myth 3   It's Performance that Really Counts!
Most men have been brainwashed into believing that their worth-whileness and masculinity are directly related to how well they perform. This whole performance attitude becomes a **real liability** during lovemaking, because our typical man is preoccupied with such things as: how long, how many, better technique, multiple positions, and so on. While he is busy thinking about and doing all this, he can't really tune in to his sensations, his emotions, and his partner, and truly enjoy himself! Furthermore, if for some reason he judges his performance as not measuring up to his expectations, he will feel anxious, angry, or dejected, and these emotional responses will spoil his pleasure and impair his performance, setting up a vicious cycle.

The truth, of course, is that all that **really** counts is sharing an enjoyable, unique, physical and emotional closeness with someone you really like or love! Anything more is just an optional extra! I don't expect you to believe this, just because I say it, but at least **try** it for a while, and see whether in fact both you and your partner actually do enjoy your lovemaking much more. See if you don't feel ever so much better when you don't have to worry about turning in a top-rating performance!

Myth 4   Good Sex Must be Super-Sex!

If you believe this, you won't enjoy lovemaking, unless it turns out to be a five-star extravaganza! You will certainly not enjoy a five-minute quickie without the trimmings when you are horny but running late for work, or going to sleep in each others arms soon after penetration, because you are both dead tired. A sexual blockbuster is great if you have the time and opportunity, but you will be much happier sexually if you lower your goals considerably, and **learn** how to enjoy basic sexual closeness.

Myth 5   Pleasurable Physical Contact Must Go on to Sex!

Men have often grown up with the idea that for them only two kinds of body contact are permissible — aggressive and sexual. This means that touching a woman without a view to sex is unacceptable. You may be surprised to know that one of the commonest serious complaints women have about men is that 'he only holds, cuddles or strokes me when he wants sex'. Women quite understandably feel resentful about this!

We all have an innate need for touching with other humans, and there is absolutely **nothing** wrong with this! By no possible stretch of the imagination is it unmanly. It can be **very** comforting sometimes simply to be held and stroked.

If you have got into the bad habit of only touching when you want sex, it will take you a while to get out of it, but you will be truly amazed at the difference it makes when you are able to engage in stroking, holding, cuddling and so on, with no sexual intent. While touching and sex remain linked together in your mind, you can't touch without **putting pressure on yourself** and your partner **to be sexual,** when perhaps this is not really desired by either of you.

Myth 6   Males Must Always be Active During Sex!

Myth 7   Men are Responsible for What Happens During Sex!

Myth 8   During Sex the Male is Responsible for his Partner's Arousal and Orgasm!

These 3 myths can be considered together, as they are closely related. Men and women are of course equal, both generally and sexually, and have the same sexual rights and responsibilities. There is

absolutely no rational reason why a man should feel responsible for everything that happens during lovemaking, as if he had to orchestrate the whole performance! What happens is surely a **shared responsibility.** Just as from time to time a woman will feel like being relatively passive sexually, so sometimes will a man, this being perfectly right and proper. Nonetheless, many men find it **very difficult** just to lie back and do nothing, passively soaking up the attentions of their partner.

During lovemaking, each partner is personally responsible for their own arousal and orgasm. It is our own responsibility to make sure that we get the kind of stimulation we wish or need, where we want it, for as long as we choose. Our only responsibility to our partner is to do our best to give her (him) what she (he) seems to want. This whole issue of responsibility is so crucially important for good lovemaking, that it will be considered again in the next chapter.

Myth 9   Sex Must Lead to Orgasm!

Myth 10   Once Started, Sex Must Continue Until Orgasms Have Been Achieved!

Myth 11   A Man and his Partner Should Reach Orgasm At the Same Time!

These orgasm myths can be considered together. It is totally inconceivable to many men that anyone could want sex but not wish or need an orgasm! However, this is a commonplace experience, particularly for women, and men as they get older. It is quite possible and perfectly normal for a person to feel a desire or need for the closeness and other emotional gratifications of sexual contact, **but not feel like having an orgasm!** You need to know that as men get older, their need for an orgasm to complete a rewarding sexual experience normally decreases. Many older men will tell you that quite often they feel horny and want intercourse, but are not really interested in having an orgasm, and there is absolutely nothing wrong with that! If you feel you or your partner simply **must** wind up having an orgasm whenever you have sex, you are putting pressure on your sexual relationship which will cause you trouble, sooner or later!

Many men erroneously believe that once sexual stimulation begins, it must continue uninterruptedly until orgasm is achieved. The notion that during lovemaking, one or both partners might like to have a rest, or listen to some music, or even have a sleep, before continuing, is just totally incomprehensible! In actual fact, you will be pleasantly surprised to discover that often **the most intense heights** of sexual arousal and pleasure are attained by lovemaking that stops and starts, rather than progresses without any pause! Try it yourself, and when it no longer seems odd, you may be in for a real treat!

The absurd and destructive simultaneous orgasm myth dies hard. Even now that most men know as an intellectual fact that only a minority of women can achieve orgasm purely from the stimulation of intercourse, they still fuss about coming with their partner! It is actually quite an improbable feat for a couple to climax together, and it is usually achieved by one partner desperately trying to hold off orgasm, while the other equally frantically tries to come sooner. If one or the other fails, there is often disappointment, frustration, a tendency to put oneself down, and the like. Bedroom olympics like this, with a win-or-lose agenda, **are a recipe for unhappiness!** The really sad fact about this whole pathetic misconception, is that truly **sharing** your partner's orgasm, by being able to observe it and experience it, is **extremely** emotionally rewarding, but **impossible** if you are coming at the same time! You are too tied up blowing your own mind to enjoy the spectacle of her doing the same thing.

Myth 12　There is No Such Thing as Sexual Monotony if You Truly Love Your Partner!

Sadly, **even love** is not sufficient to keep your sex life exciting and stimulating! It will only remain this way if you keep working at it, using your joint erotic imaginations to the full. After the initial excitement and novelty of getting to know each other wears off, many couples find that their lovemaking gradually becomes something of a predictable routine, which never varies very much. **Sexual monotony** has then set in. Some seek to rekindle sexual excitement with a different partner, others erroneously believe the situation is an inevitable consequence of ageing, leading often to them ultimately giving up on sex altogether. As the excitement of lovemaking decreases, often so does a man's ability to get a hard-on, simply because he is just not getting adequately mentally aroused!

The remedy is obvious enough — revamp your sex life! Get out of your sexual rut! You will be pleasantly surprised with the results if you **both** make the effort!

How to Overcome the Destructive Effects of Sexual Myths

This is not easy, but it is **absolutely** essential, and will take you some considerable time! You certainly won't make **any** progress at all just by being aware of the stupidity of these myths. **The only practical way to change these faulty attitudes is to alter your behaviour,** to get in there and actively **do** something relevant! Get stuck into the following exercises **before** you read on!

1. Go through the myths listed in this chapter, and **write down** those which you feel have some effect on you.
2. For each myth affecting you, do the following:
    a. **Write down** all the numerous practical ways in which this myth has caused problems or difficulties for you. Illustrate each with an **actual example,** from your past, which you should also **write down.**
    b. **Write down** all the reasons you can think of why the myth and its consequences are ridiculous and destructive. Give this some real thought, and take your time.
    c. If at all possible, discuss **in detail** what you have done in a. and b. with your partner.
3. Rewrite your entire list of personally relevant myths, but now in **logical rational terms.** For example, if a relevant myth affecting you is this: 'During sex the male is responsible for his partner's arousal and orgasm', re-write it, something like this: 'I am not responsible for my partner's arousal and orgasm — she is! My only responsibility to her is to do my best to give her what she lets me know she wants'.
4. Read this list of logically re-written myths, out loud, once a day, **with feeling.** Continue doing this until you have completely finished working on your erection problem!
5. For each personally relevant myth, work out and **write down** some actual corrective behaviours, or things **to do** to help you overcome the destructive effects of the myth. For example, take

the myth 'pleasurable physical contact must go on to sex'. Your corrective behaviours might involve things such as:

a. 'I will make a deliberate effort to stroke, cuddle and touch my partner as often as I can, in situations where there is no possibility of sex, such as just before I leave for work, when we go out together, while driving together and so on.'

b. 'I will frequently engage in deliberate gentle sexual touching, such as breast and genital fondling and stroking, but without following through and making love. I will do this sometimes when we watch TV together alone, sometimes when we go to bed, sometimes when we have a brief spontaneous cuddle around the house. Even if I then feel like following through, I will deliberately stop myself'.

6. Make a definite **ongoing** effort to carry out your personal corrective behaviours **as often as possible.** You will find that it is best to hammer away repeatedly at the corrective behaviours directed at **only one myth at a time,** rather than several or the whole lot. When you feel you have reasonably changed a particular faulty attitude, then and only then, have a crack at your corrective exercises directed at the next myth you wish to tackle.

A Few Important Practical Tips

1. Do these exercises **thoroughly** — don't rush through them! It will take some considerable time, but it is time very well spent. Remember, your future sexual happiness is at stake!

2. A little done often is better than trying to do everything in one long session.

3. When you have finished each written exercise, put it away for a few days, then go through it again, to see if you have any new ideas about it.

4. Don't make the mistake of persuading yourself that you will read the whole book first, then come back and do these exercises! To get the maximum benefit, you simply **must** do the necessary exercises **as you come to them!**

5. Share as much as possible of what you are doing with your partner. **The more she is involved and understands, the easier everything will be for you!**

Chapter 6

YOUR CONDITIONS OR REQUIREMENTS FOR BEING SEXUALLY RESPONSIVE

This is one of the most critically important chapters in this book!

Pay great attention to it!

One of the most ridiculous misconceptions men have about their sexual functioning is the idea that they should be able to get an erection whenever they want one, under any circumstances! This has been considered in the previous chapter, and hopefully by now you can see how totally idiotic this notion is! The hard facts are almost the exact opposite! **No man has any rational grounds for expecting to be sexually responsive and able to erect adequately, unless his own personal conditions or requirements for being sexually responsive are reasonably met!**

When you are young, often your sexual nervous system is so excitable, that the least little thing will lead to an erection. This often occurs and persists in an embarrassing manner, even when the last thing you want is a hard-on! This common observation unfortunately supports the myth already picked up from one's equally sexually ignorant and inexperienced friends, that a real man can get an erection whenever he wants, no matter what. It doesn't take too many years into maturity however, for men to be confronted with the fallacy of this crazy idea, because as we get older, our erectile mechanism becomes much less excitable. Sooner or later we simply have to accept the notion that we cannot get it up, unless we have some basic things going for us — in other words, unless our conditions or requirements for being sexually responsive are met. **The older we get, the more crucial it becomes for us to pay attention to these conditions!**

What Does this Concept of Necessary Conditions Actually Mean?

A condition is essentially anything that can affect your ability to respond sexually. In other words, it is something the presence or absence of which makes it easier for you to respond. It may be something in you, in your partner, in your relationship, or in your environment.

What are Your Conditions for Being Sexually Responsive?

As a rule, these are a personal, individual matter, although some are applicable to most men. These general conditions will now be described.

1. Not being too tired! If you are tired, you have no rational grounds for expecting to be sexually responsive.
2. Absence of significant physical discomfort! If you have a nasty headache, or your bad back is playing up and causing a lot of pain, or if you are in any other way significantly uncomfortable, it is ridiculous to expect your erectile mechanism to function normally.
3. Absence of emotional 'uptightness'! If you are feeling guilty, frustrated, angry, worried, or miserable and down in the dumps, do not expect to be able to get it up, since these emotional states can have a very powerful inhibiting effect on your erection mechanism.
4. Presence of sexual drive or interest! If for some reason you are not particularly interested in sex at any given time, you will be pushing your luck if you expect to be able to erect normally.

Although it may at first seem hard to believe, **many men think they are interested in sex, when they really aren't.** This is because they rely on the situation they are in, rather than their own feelings, to define interest. If their situation is one they have learned to label as sexy, such as being with an attractive woman who wants sex, they often **assume** they are interested, because they feel they should be!

Note that if your partner is sexually interested, but you are not in the mood for shared lovemaking, there is absolutely no reason why you can't simply let her know how you feel, and then offer to pleasure her, and bring her to orgasm by some form of stimulation other than intercourse. There is no law that says you have to be actively involved and erect whenever you are in a sexual situation! It is of course simply basic good sexual manners, to offer your partner sexual tension relief if she is aroused and you are not in the mood. Hopefully she will reciprocate when the situation is reversed.

5. Presence of interest in or attraction to your partner! If you are not interested in or attracted to your partner, even if you are feeling aroused, what on earth are you doing making love with her? On what vaguely rational grounds can you possibly expect to get a hard-on? Asking your penis to perform under these circumstances is almost an insult to it!

6. Absence of concern about your own sexual performance! If you are concerned about (or thinking about) how well or otherwise you will perform, or about what your partner will think of your lovemaking, you are activating one of the most powerful and destructive inhibitors of erection, and you have no sensible grounds for even hoping to get it up!

7. Absence of tension in your relationship with your partner! If, when you want intercourse, you are feeling negative towards your partner, your penis will probably react as though it feels exactly the same way! It may in fact take some time after your negative feelings have been overcome, before it is able to respond as you would wish! For example, you cannot logically expect to be normally responsive 5 minutes after an argument with your partner has been resolved.

8. Absence of unhelpful thoughts! Even if you are not emotionally uptight, if some unresolved problem or issue from the day is still ticking over in your mind, you may find your penis will not function properly. If your penis is to do the right thing by you, it expects you to do the right thing by it — in other words, that you concentrate on the sensual and erotic aspects of the sexual situation. You simply can't do this adequately if your mind is elsewhere!

9. Presence of adequate mental and physical stimulation! Especially as you get a bit older, you cannot expect to get a hard-on just because you happen to be interested and in a sexual situation with your partner. Particularly if lovemaking has become a fairly stereotyped ritual, no matter how much you love your partner, and how attractive you find her, you may not find the sexual situation stimulating or arousing enough to generate an adequate erection. You may need **not just** more mental stimulation and excitement, but more direct penile manipulation as well.

10. Presence of an adequate physical environment! Are you free from the possibility of interruption? Do other people nearby know what you are doing or can they hear you? Are you expecting the phone to go at any moment? Are you too cold or too hot? Common sense dictates that lovemaking needs to occur in an adequate environment, without which it is unreasonable and stupid to expect your penis to behave as you would wish!

11. Absence of too much alcohol (or some other sedative drugs)! Remember, the amount of alcohol in your blood which is required to impair your ability to get it up is **very variable from man to man!** Some men are adversely affected by even small amounts. In general, men with erection problems should be very careful indeed with their alcohol consumption! **It is impossible to emphasize this too strongly!**

Many men I have counselled have found it hard to accept their need to pay attention to some of these conditions, arguing that **previously** they have been able to erect adequately, despite the absence of these requirements. Others cite people known to them, who can (or allege they can!) perform under any circumstances,

no matter how adverse. It is true, that there are a few men whose
ability to get it up seems largely unaffected by their emotional or
physical state — as if somehow their penis was insulated from their
feelings. You might envy this ability, but **not logically,** because more
often than not, such men pay a terrible price for this ability — they
are unable to experience much real pleasure during lovemaking.

We men **must understand and accept** that getting older
produces changes in our pattern of sexual responsiveness, and one
crucial change is that we simply have to begin paying attention
to our conditions for being sexually responsive! This becomes
progressively more important as we get older!

The fact that perhaps previously you could ignore many conditions,
and still get it up, certainly does not mean you can keep on ignoring
them! You just have to accept the fact that sooner or later, you and
every other man, are going to be **forced** to pay attention to your
conditions, **whether you like it or not!**

Many men who have been reared on a solid diet of sexual myths,
from which few of us can escape, feel that having conditions for being
responsive is a sign of weakness or inadequacy, unmanly, feminine
and so on. They find the idea of conditions almost repugnant! If this
is how you feel, you had better start working on changing these
ridiculous attitudes, or **in the long run you will pay a terrible price**
(in unhappiness) for your folly! I can assure you that you will have
much more success changing your irrational beliefs, than you will
have trying to alter your conditions for erecting adequately!

Specific Personal Conditions or Requirements

Over and above the **general** issues already discussed, many men
have personal requirements, as one would expect, since we are all
unique individuals with different needs, tastes and interests. This is
seen most graphically in men who have what is called a sexual fetish,
and who must have their particular fetish present in order to be
potent. For example, this might involve a specific environment or
garment. You might regard such peculiar requirements as ridiculous,
or even a bit kinky, but they are harmless, and **much** easier to live
with than to change, and anyway, **what is wrong with being a
little different?**

Exercises for Working Out Your Conditions

When you have privacy, and are not tired or preoccupied, sit down with paper and pen nearby, and with your eyes closed, think of the most recent sexual experience you can remember, which you found very satisfying, **and where you had no erection problems.** Run through the whole encounter in your mind, from the very earliest stages to the end. When you have done this, write down **all** the factors you can think of, that contributed to such a successful outcome — in yourself, your partner, your relationship and in the general environment. When you have finished as best you can, run through the **general** conditions discussed in this chapter, and see whether they too applied — if so, add them to your list.

If you have not had an exciting and successful sexual encounter which you can recall, sit back and imagine in detail a make-believe, ideal encounter, then work out some of your conditions as above.

Next, run through in your mind, the worst, most unsatisfactory sexual encounter you can remember, using this to work out more of your conditions, exactly as described above. When you have finished, run through my list of general conditions, and see how they applied to that unsatisfactory encounter. Write down what you have learned.

When you have done both these exercises, see if you can think of anything else at all which **does** or **could** possibly affect, for better or worse, the pleasure or satisfaction you would experience in a sexual encounter. Write these down. Remember, a condition is basically absolutely anything that affects your ability to respond sexually!

When you have run out of fresh ideas about your conditions, see if you can discuss everything you have written down with your partner. Make sure she gets you to clarify everything, so that she knows **exactly** what you mean! **Avoid communicating with her in generalities — be absolutely specific!** For example, saying: 'I need adequate penile stimulation', is **far too general**. This needs to be **expanded considerably** — where? precisely how? when? for how long? and so on.

If you don't have a partner with whom you can discuss these issues, **pretend you are your partner,** and ask yourself the sort of questions a real partner would ask, to clarify **precisely** what you mean.

When all this has been done, summarize everything you have learned about yourself from this chapter and the exercises. In other words, write down your definitive list of your conditions for being adequately sexually responsive! Make sure they are written in **absolutely practical terms,** not generalities. **Exactly** what you need must be **crystal clear!**

Check that your list contains as a condition something like this: 'Knowing and accepting that an erection is not in any way necessary for satisfactory and successful lovemaking'. This is **absolutely essential** if you have had erection problems!

Keep your final list somewhere handy, so that you can read it through carefully, **out loud and with feeling,** once daily, **for the remainder of the time you are working on overcoming your erectile problem!**

With the passage of time, you will probably find that your 'final' list grows, as you become increasingly aware of all the various additional factors which affect your sexual behaviour!

If you can, explain to as many friends and acquaintances as possible, both male and female, the general issue of conditions for being sexually responsive. Counter any argument, as I have tried to do in this book. By teaching others, you are impressing these very important notions much more firmly into your own mind, and this will help you even more.

Your Sexual Rights and Responsibilities

Men and women are equals, generally and sexually. This means that they have the same sexual rights and responsibilities. An **important requirement** for good lovemaking is that you are able to easily, comfortably and appropriately exercise your sexual rights and responsibilities!

Contrary to the erroneous views held by many men and women, a man is **not** responsible for his partner's arousal and ultimate orgasm — these are **her** responsibility! As a man, **your only responsibility to your partner** is to do your best to give her the kind of stimulation she desires on any particular occasion. If she doesn't clearly communicate her needs and wishes, and therefore misses the boat, that is **her problem** and **her responsibility, not yours!** The same of course applies in reverse — if you do not let her know **exactly** what you would like, what kind of stimulation you need, and so on, then you can only blame yourself if your needs are not met and in consequence you do not become adequately aroused!

Of course, this is not to say that each partner must always do exactly what the other wishes! Some forms of stimulation enjoyed by one may be unacceptable to the other, and there is certainly no law stating that you have to do something you find unacceptable! If there is conflict between you and your partner over performing some kind of sexual behaviour, discuss the issues when you are **not** in a sexual situation, and see if you can come to understand each other's point of view, and then perhaps agree to some mutually acceptable compromise.

As an equal partner in a sexual relationship, you have certain rights, which are exactly the same as those of your partner. You have the right to ask for or to initiate lovemaking — she of course has the right to decline — and vice versa. You have the right to ask for any particular form of stimulation or activity you desire, including sexual contact without orgasm or without intercourse. You have a right during lovemaking to cease personal participation if you no longer feel like it — of course, hopefully you would then offer to relieve your partner's sexual tension by manipulating her to orgasm, should she desire this. You also have a right to express how you feel about any aspect of lovemaking. However, be **very gentle** if ever you have to say **anything even vaguely critical** about your partner's lovemaking! **All humans are extremely vulnerable to even minor criticism of their sexual prowess!** Some hints on improving your sexual communication are offered in appendix 11.

You might now say that you accept the fact of your rights, but would find it difficult or impossible to actually exercise them with a partner. In other words, you just could not say the appropriate things to her, even though you know you have every right to do so. Apart from working to improve your general sexual communication, a simple way to overcome this difficulty is repeatedly to practise saying the kinds of things you would find difficult to say to her, into a tape recorder. Listen to the playback, and give yourself constructive criticism and appropriate praise. Repeat one particular problem statement over and over again, varying it just a little each time, until you feel satisfied with the way you sound. Practising frequently, but for only a few minutes at a time, works best. Five minutes is the **maximum** useful period for this kind of rehearsal.

If you practise in this way on a daily basis, it should only take a few weeks until you feel comfortable enough to say this kind of thing with a partner.

Please note: I am **not** in any way suggesting that you rehearse or memorize specific lines, to be trotted out at some future date! You are instead rehearsing a general skill, and you will ultimately find that under the appropriate sexual circumstances, you will say whatever you wish to communicate, easily, comfortably and spontaneously.

Now, do yourself some favours!

1. Do not read any further, or do any other exercises, until you have thoroughly done everything that I have asked you to do in this chapter.
2. Read **out loud** to yourself, **with feeling,** your final list of specific conditions, **every day,** until your problem is ancient history!
3. **Never** get into a sexual situation where there is any expectation that you will be sexually responsive, **unless most of your personal conditions are adequately met!** Explain why, to your partner, **without any apology.** She will clearly understand, since women from even young adulthood, are even more bound by their sexual conditions than we men.

Chapter 7

HOW DO YOU KNOW YOU HAVE A PROBLEM OF IMPOTENCE?

Believe it or not, this can be a difficult question to answer! Most men **occasionally** have difficulty getting an erection when they would like one, or cannot get one at all, or may obtain an erection, but be unable to maintain it. This is all perfectly normal and **such men do not have a problem of impotence!** This term has the clear implication that the difficulty in obtaining or maintaining an adequate erection occurs **frequently** or **all the time!**

What is an Adequate Erection?

Since the only function of an erection is to enable penetration of one's partner, an adequate erection is one which is firm enough to achieve this. A relatively loose vagina can be penetrated by a less firm penis than a tight vagina, and some women are more skilful than others at facilitating penetration by a less than fully erect penis, so just what constitutes an adequate erection is influenced by **both partners.**

What then is Impotence?

For practical purposes this term refers to usual or habitual difficulty in erecting to a degree adequate for penetration of one's sexual partner, or to usual or habitual difficulty in maintaining an erection adequate for thrusting into one's partner until ejaculation occurs.

Is there a Better Term than Impotence?

Because of popular usage, the word impotence has all kinds of negative connotations, such as worthless, inadequate, unmanly and so on, and these add greatly to the problems and misery of affected men. A better, more meaningful term, is 'erectile dysfunction', which is relatively free of negative associations.

Types of Erection Problems

Some men have difficulty getting hard enough for penetration. Others have no great problem getting hard, but they cannot then maintain the erection. A man may have no problems getting a normal enough erection in one situation, but be unable to do so in another. For example, he may have no problems erecting in private masturbation, but be unable to erect during sexual contact with a partner, or he may erect without difficulty with one partner, but not with another.

Usually, the lack of hardness affects the whole penis, but sometimes only a portion of it is affected. For example, the base of the penis may become quite firm, but the end be too soft for penetration — this is sometimes referred to as 'end wobble'.

Sometimes one side of the penis erects normally or reasonably normally, but the other does not, causing the penis to bend towards the abnormal side during erection.

Some medical writers distinguish between 'acute situational' and 'chronic' impotence. The first variety occurs when a man with no prior history of erection problems, finds himself **suddenly** unable to erect adequately or unable to maintain an adequate erection, because of stress, anxiety, fatigue, intoxication with alcohol and so on. He then worries about his sexual performance so much that the erection problem continues, despite the removal of the adverse circumstances which caused it on the first occasion. Chronic impotence describes a long-standing or recurrent problem with erections.

The practical importance of knowing the particular type of impotence involved, lies in what it may tell about the causes of the problem, and how to overcome it.

Misconceptions About the Meaning of the Term Impotence

Some men fear they are becoming impotent because for one reason or another their sexual drive or interest has decreased, even though they have no problem getting and keeping an erection when they wish to have sex. This is **not** impotence but a problem of decreased sexual drive, which is a **completely separate** issue.

Some men have in the past often had intercourse a second time in a single session of lovemaking, after a brief rest following their first ejaculation. When with increasing age they find they can no longer erect a second time, they may feel they are becoming impotent, even though there are absolutely no problems getting and keeping an erection the first time around. Such men do **not** have a problem of impotence — they simply have quite unrealistic expectations of themselves!

The normal changes to the process of erection associated with ageing (chapter 4) do **not** indicate the presence of a problem, although many men feel they have a potency difficulty because of these changes, and their practical consequences.

Unfortunately, in the medical literature on sexual problems in the past, the term impotence has been used loosely to describe other problems, for example, too rapid ejaculation or difficulty ejaculating. These have **nothing** to do with impotence, which refers **only** to erection problems!

Chapter 8

WHAT YOU NEED TO KNOW ABOUT THE CAUSES OF IMPOTENCE

Most frequently, erection problems are due not to one single cause, but to a variety of factors acting together, no one of these by itself being responsible for the problem.

Contributory causes can for convenience be divided into 4 groups:
1. 'constitutional vulnerability';
2. chemical agents;
3. physical diseases or abnormalities;
4. psychological factors.

Constitutional Vulnerability

Most of us, if stressed enough, will develop some physical symptom or symptoms, such as diarrhoea, tension headaches, frequent urination and so on. Usually we develop the same physical symptoms quite predictably if we are sufficiently stressed. For example, some men **always** get diarrhoea — for them, their bowel is in some way particularly susceptible to the effects of stress.

It would appear that some men's erection mechanism is especially vulnerable to stress, which then tends to induce impotence. The exact reason for this particular sensitivity is not known, but it is in some way built into the individual's makeup. Such men are said to have a 'constitutional vulnerability' to erection problems, just as others have a constitutional vulnerability to diarrhoea. Nothing can be done to alter a constitutional vulnerability to erection problems, but a man with such a predisposition can do much to prevent it becoming activated by stress, as will be discussed later.

Chemical Agents as Contributory Causes of Impotence

Some chemicals used in industry and agriculture, and many drugs prescribed by doctors, can **contribute** to the development and maintenance of impotence. However, the commonest chemical contributions to impotence come from **alcohol** and **nicotine** (from smoking).

If a man with an erectile problem is exposed to particular chemicals in his work or hobbies, he could check with a government or university department of occupational health to find out whether the agents concerned could possibly have any effect on erections. If they could, appropriate measures to prevent such exposure are indicated. In actual fact however, very few industrial chemicals to which men are exposed are known to contribute to erection problems.

Many prescribed drugs are known to induce erection problems in some men. No drug always causes impotence in every man exposed to the doses used in medicine. In fact, with most drugs capable of inducing impotence, this side effect occurs in **only a small percentage of men** taking it! Why this occurs is often not well understood, but sometimes it is due to the drug **adding to the effect of another pre-existing contributory factor,** the combination leading to impotence. Some people simply appear to be more susceptible to this side effect. The drugs known to induce impotence at least occasionally are many and varied, and include some (but certainly not all) blood pressure-lowering drugs, tranquillizers and antidepressants. **If you are taking any drug, and have an erection problem, check with your doctor as to whether or not it has ever been found to contribute to impotence!** If he doesn't know, he can look up its published side effects or contact the drug company who market the drug, who would certainly know. You must understand clearly however, that just because a drug you are taking can **sometimes** contribute to impotence, this does **not** in any way mean it is involved in **your** erection problem! The only way to be sure, is to stop the drug (if that is medically advisable, which only your doctor can decide), or change it to one which will give you the same benefit, but hopefully not contribute to impotence.

Alcohol consumed in sufficiently large quantities will interfere with any man's erectile capacity, but some men are particularly susceptible to the erection-inhibiting effect of alcohol, and require only a very small quantity to induce impotence. Long continued excessive alcohol consumption can contribute to impotence by causing damage to a variety of body structures affecting the erectile process.

In some men, smoking can be shown to decrease the amount of blood flowing into the penis, and this may be a critical factor in precipitating impotence. The nicotine content is believed to be responsible for this effect. Long-continued smoking is one factor clearly contributing to a disease of arteries (atherosclerosis) leading to them narrowing or becoming blocked, and decreased blood flow into the penis resulting from this may not improve when smoking is ceased. There is no doubt however, that **some** smokers have their impotence reversed or alleviated when they cease smoking, although it can take as long as 3 months to achieve the maximum benefit which will then result. **Any impotent man who smokes is very well advised to give up smoking completely!**

Physical Diseases or Abnormalities as Contributory Causes of Impotence

A very large number of physical conditions can contribute to erectile difficulties. The commonest appear to be diseases or disorders interfering with blood flow into the penis, or resulting in blood draining out of the penis too rapidly. Diabetes is another disorder commonly contributing to erectile problems. It must be clearly understood however, that **usually a majority of men suffering from a particular disease sometimes capable of inducing impotence, have absolutely no erectile problems at all at any stage!** Just because an impotent man suffers from a disease which can sometimes induce impotence, for example diabetes, does **not** mean that his problem is necessarily due to that disease. Other factors may be responsible, or add to the effects of that disease, to produce the symptom of impotence. Even if in a particular case it can be shown that a disease such as diabetes actually **is** a factor contributing to impotence, **this does not in any way mean that the impotence cannot be overcome,** even though the effects of the disease may be irreversible. **Often enough in clinical practice it is quite possible to restore adequate potency despite considerable contributions to the problem from irreversible physical diseases!**

A small number of diseases contributing to impotence are, or can become, quite serious left untreated, and need medical attention. Ways of recognizing this possibility will be discussed later.

Psychological Factors Contributing to Impotence

For convenience, these can be divided into 'personal' and 'relationship' influences.

Personal Issues

The single most important psychological factor contributing to impotence is anxiety, which is a **very powerful** inhibitor of the erection mechanism. Anxiety of almost **any cause** can do the trick! Once a man has experienced an episode of impotence, he will very often be anxious about it happening again. This anxiety about possibly being impotent, is sometimes called 'performance anxiety'.

Performance anxiety is enormously important, and **grossly destructive!** For example, I have seen many men who suffered a single episode of impotence, simply due to fatigue or too much alcohol, who then worried so much about whether or not they would get an erection, that they became chronically impotent, even though the original cause of the problem no longer existed!

If you are anxious, it is very often because you are thinking thoughts which make you anxious! Anxiety-generating thoughts when you are in a sexual situation, are usually there because you have irrational beliefs about various aspects of sex, based on the myths discussed in chapter 5. Alternatively, anxiety-producing thoughts may be about an unwanted pregnancy resulting, being discovered, catching venereal disease, ejaculating too quickly, and so on.

A man concerned about getting an erection almost always makes the mistake of **actively trying** to get it up, by contracting his pelvic muscles, and other manoeuvres. This is just about **the worst thing he could do, because the harder he tries, usually the more difficult it will be to erect!**

Stress can be an important factor contributing to impotence, and may operate in a variety of ways. It can make you tense and anxious, or preoccupied, so that your 'conditions' for erecting are not met. Chronic stress can be debilitating, so that you are generally run down, this once again interfering with your necessary conditions. In some men, stress rather specifically interferes with erections, because of their constitutional vulnerability, as discussed earlier.

Anger, guilt, shame, unhappiness, disgust, jealousy and other negative emotions, can interfere with your ability to erect, just as anxiety does. It doesn't seem to much matter what causes you to be angry, guilty and so on, as the emotions themselves often appear to be able to block erections, more or less regardless of their cause.

If you have what is technically called a 'depressive illness', this may render you impotent. The whole issue is somewhat complex, because **you do not have to actually feel particularly depressed to have this ailment!** The recognition of this very common psychological disorder is discussed in chapter 10. Potency is often restored simply by treating this illness.

A man's upbringing can predispose him to the future development of erection problems, by making him vulnerable to certain situations. For example, if as a young lad, he was made to feel guilty about masturbation, and severely punished for it by his mother, he may well be predisposed to feeling guilty about sex, and anxious about being accepted and loved by a woman if he is sexual. If, as an adult, something relatively trivial happens in his sexual relationship with his partner, such as an innocent rejection, because she is simply too tired, this may activate irrational guilt and anxiety, which subsequently interferes with his potency.

Specific traumatic events can sometimes bring on erection problems. For example, one young man became completely impotent overnight, when he found out that his wife had been having an affair. Even when the couple had sorted out the situation, and made a new commitment to each other, total impotence persisted. He reported that now, when he was making love with his wife, he could not stop himself thinking about her having intercourse with her former lover, these thoughts upsetting him greatly. This very effectively completely blocked his erection mechanism.

In Summary
1. Anxiety of almost any cause, but especially about sexual performance, is the commonest personal psychological factor contributing to the development and/or maintenance of impotence.
2. Anxiety in the sexual situation is often due to unhelpful thoughts, most often based on destructive sexual myths.
3. Trying to **make** an erection occur causes the whole process to become much more difficult, or even impossible.
4. Stress can interfere with erectile ability.
5. Anger, guilt, shame, unhappiness, disgust and jealousy can inhibit erections, more or less regardless of their cause.
6. A common psychological ailment, often inducing impotence, is a depressive illness.
7. Your upbringing can predispose you to inappropriate anxiety, guilt and so on, and thus to impotence.
8. Traumatic events, and their consequences, can sometimes bring on and maintain impotence.

Relationship Issues

If his relationship with his partner is in poor shape, a man may not be able to erect adequately with her, ultimately **because not enough of his conditions for being responsive are met!** Of course, sometimes he may not really want to get it up with a partner with whom he is angry, as a way of **punishing** her, even though he may selfrighteously conceal this motive from himself!

It is, of course, perfectly obvious that any angry or critical response to your difficulty from your partner, will make it even harder to erect adequately. However, **even the occasional quite unavoidable non-verbal reaction of disappointment or concern from a truly loving, caring and accepting partner, will tend to increase your anxiety about your erection problem, thereby making it worse!**

A not uncommon partner response to impotence, which is intended to be **supportive,** but unfortunately often proves to be unhelpful, goes like this:

'Sweetheart, don't worry about it — it doesn't concern me. Let's just quit and go to sleep'.

This sounds reassuring, and is indeed intended to be so. However, the impotent man very often erroneously reads into this the following message:

'No fuss, but no erection, no sex'.

Since most men, at some level, subscribe to the view that sex is not possible without an erection, it is easy to see how their misinterpretation of their partner's message in fact puts even more pressure on them, increasing the self-inflicted need to perform.

The **ideal** partner response, of course, is this:

'It doesn't make the slightest difference to me whether you erect adequately or not: we are still making love, which is what it's all about and what I most enjoy, so let's just carry on, regardless'. This acts to effectively decrease performance concerns.

Another response, intended to be loving and helpful, but also often backfiring, goes like this:

The partner, during lovemaking, goes to great lengths to help her man get an erection, hammering away at stimulating the penis one way or the other, with a real vengeance, often for lengthy periods of time. An equally unhelpful variation on this same theme, is her **repeatedly** coming back to attempting to manipulate the penis to erection. Unfortunately, the impotent man sees his partner as **actively trying to make him erect,** which increases the pressure on getting an erection, making the problem worse.

Ideally, on any particular occasion, your partner will be trying to achieve the difficult and delicate balance between providing you with adequate physical genital stimulation on the one hand, and on the other, being seen as not caring about whether or not an erection adequate for penetration is achieved.

Other occasional psychological contributions by the partner to the various factors adding together to produce impotence, or perpetuating it, include:

1. Poor communication, during lovemaking, or about the erectile problem.
2. Lack of knowledge about proper erotic technique.
3. Lack of knowledge about the effects of ageing and how to compensate for these.
4. Adherence to behaviour controlled by sexual myths, such as 'it's all up to the man', and so on.
5. Lack of genuine interest in sexual relating.

Certain relationship issues are so crucially important in treatment, that they will be considered again in different contexts, particularly in chapters 9 and 10.

Chapter 9

HOW DO MEN AND WOMEN REACT TO IMPOTENCE?

Many men see impotence as a total personal disaster. This is largely because their self-image depends on performance, and their concept of themselves as a proper man hinges on their sexual capability. They may react with anxiety, depression or anger, all of which then usually make the erection problem **much worse.** In a sexual situation, men with erection difficulties are usually working at trying to **make** an erection occur; these active efforts simply decrease the possibility of an adequate erection being achieved. They may avoid sexual situations as they anticipate humiliation, and try to push their sexual feelings and needs out of their minds. This avoidance once again makes the erection problem worse. Severe depression may develop and suicide has occurred. Some drown their misery in alcohol.

A few men appear just to accept the problem without distress, especially if they are older and believe impotence is an inevitable consequence of increasing age. Provided any involved partner expresses no concern, the individual or couple may then live out their life without any form of sexual expression.

Some couples work out a pattern of mutually satisfying sexual contact based on loveplay and mutual manipulation to orgasm.

One's professional experience suggests that a majority of men are really extremely worried about their difficulty, however well this concern may be concealed from others, including partners, and even from themselves!

While impotence is certainly no blessing, there is absolutely no rational reason why it should generate the strong emotional reactions described, or even interfere very much with satisfactory lovemaking! When it does, this is largely because of the malignant and destructive effects of the widespread myths about sexual functioning, described in chapter 5.

Women in general are usually much less concerned about impotence than their male partners, although one sees occasional exceptions. Commonly, when persistent impotence first occurs in their partner, women begin to wonder whether there is in fact something wrong with **them!** Are they still sexually attractive to him? Does he still love her? Is their own sexual performance adequate? Ideally, and in a truly good relationship, the partner of an impotent man will be supportive of him and his concerns about the problem. She will indicate that intercourse is not the be all and end all, and that what is most important to her, is the closeness and tenderness of sexual relating, which continues to be possible and desired. However, in even the very best relationships, when the woman has genuinely enjoyed intercourse with her partner, it is almost impossible for her to avoid betraying some anxiety, disappointment or frustration, at least occasionally. Unfortunately, even these perfectly understandable responses tend to aggravate the man's concern over his erectile problem, making it worse. A woman's enthusiastic efforts to **make** an erection occur have the same effect.

Unfortunately, some couples fail to discuss the problem openly together, because of embarrassment or a woman's fear of hurting her partner's feelings. This may result in the couple unwillingly colluding to completely give up on any form of sexual expression together.

Sadly, a few women react to the erectile difficulties of their partner angrily and critically, as though he were deliberately depriving them of something to which they feel entitled. Such partner reactions enormously compound the man's difficulties and make potency infinitely more difficult to regain. Such extreme reactions usually indicate that the couple's relationship is basically of poor quality.

Some women, who deep down have never really been very interested in sex, or much enjoyed it, may actually at some level almost welcome their partner's impotence, because now they have an opportunity to avoid something which previously they have merely gone along with for their partner's sake, out of love for him.

In some, fortunately rare but particularly unhealthy, relationships it may very well actually suit the woman to have her husband impotent. This is not simply because she doesn't enjoy sex, but mainly because she has an irrational need to control him, and impotence gives her a very effective way of doing this. Because he feels guilty about what he sees as his inadequacy, and about not being able to give his wife what he believes she wants, he is very ready to go along with whatever she wishes as a way of trying to make things up to her. Because he fears that she may otherwise reject him, or leave him, he works hard at pleasing her, and before long, his partner has complete control over him, calling all the shots. A woman like this often tends to act like a martyr about sex, but when one tries to treat her partner's impotence, threatening to get him out from under her thumb, she often actively sabotages the whole treatment effort. Over the years I have developed a clinical rule which has served me extremely well — the more vigorously and often a woman complains about her man's impotence, the more likely it is that at some level she really needs to have him impotent! Her complaining keeps him feeling guilty, and she controls him by exploiting his problem.

Sometimes one sees a man and his partner who appear genuinely concerned about his impotence, stating that apart from this difficulty, their relationship is absolutely perfect. However, when one gets to know the couple better and observes their interaction, it becomes obvious that the relationship is really in poor shape, but that neither partner can face up to this awful truth. The couple collude together to perpetuate the myth that the impotence is their only problem. It then becomes something they both 'need', because without this face-saving explanation for their acknowledged difficulties, they would have to face up to the ugly fact that they lacked the personal resources to make their relationship really work. Needless to say, impotence in this setting will not respond to any treatment measures unless the more basic relationship problems are exposed, acknowledged and somehow resolved.

Some important generalizations based on clinical experience can now be offered. Firstly, most emotional reactions a man can develop to his impotence will make it worse. Secondly, nearly every reaction a partner can show (except that of complete acceptance **and** the unfaltering pursuit of lovemaking using non-intercourse techniques), will tend ultimately to aggravate impotence. Finally, by far the most important psychological factor determining the outcome of the treatment of impotence, is the quality of the relationship with the partner. It is truly amazing how often even potency problems substantially contributed to by irreversible physical changes, can be overcome with the assistance of a truly loving, caring and cooperative partner!

If you don't have a partner, please do not in any way interpret this last statement as meaning that without one, you cannot overcome your problem, as this is certainly not true! It is a fact, however, that if you do have a partner, **and** she is other than loving, caring and truly cooperative, your task will be much more difficult!

It should by now be crystal clear that when a man with erectile difficulties has a partner, it is not just **his** problem, but **their** problem, since his partner's genital structure, erotic skill and psychological reactions to the difficulty, heavily influence his erectile performance. A logical consequence of this insight is that **when an impotent man has a partner, she simply must be actively involved in any treatment programme!** Without her willing participation and cooperation, there are limitations on what any therapist or treatment can achieve. If she is actively uncooperative, her partner has little chance of again being potent with her, until and unless her attitudes and behaviour can be modified.

Chapter 10

HOW TO EVALUATE YOUR PROBLEM AND PREPARE FOR DIRECT TREATMENT OF YOUR IMPOTENCE

Self-Evaluation

You must realize that there are important limitations on just how far you can go in working out the various factors contributing to your difficulty. This is true, even if you have a good deal of medical and psychological knowledge, since we are all blind to many aspects of our particular situation, because we are too close to it. Nonetheless, you can realistically aim to sort out some of the main issues and decide when you may need outside help.

Using the headings discussed in chapter 8 as a guide to the cause of impotence, let us systematically check you out.

Constitutional Vulnerability

Is there evidence from your past history that your penis is especially susceptible to stressful events? If so, you must be very careful to minimize stress in your life as best possible, and to overcome the adverse effects of stress by regular relaxation, as described in appendix 5. You must also pay even more careful attention than other men to making sure your conditions for being sexually responsive (chapter 6), are met!

Chemical Factors

Are you exposed to any chemicals at work or in your hobbies? Are you taking any medications, prescribed or over-the-counter? If so, check them out as suggested in chapter 8.

If you are a smoker, you should make every effort to stop completely!

If you have difficulty, check with your family physician or local health department for advice about the kinds of assistance available. Don't expect stopping smoking to have an immediate beneficial effect on your erection problem — it may take months for any benefit to be apparent.

If you use **alcohol,** it is well worthwhile experimenting to see whether it is aggravating your problem, by stopping **completely** for at least a month. If you find it difficult to stop drinking completely, you may have a drinking problem, and you should seek guidance as to whether or not you do, and if so, how you can overcome it. A good family physician will be able to help here.

Physical Diseases or Abnormalities

These present a real problem in self-evaluation. There is no doubt that it would be desirable for you to have a full head-to-toes medical examination from your doctor. Because this is very time consuming, you might have to arrange a special long appointment. Remember however, that **an 'all-clear' finding from a competently performed general physical examination does not in any way mean there are no physical factors contributing to your erection problem!** Some relevant disorders can **only** be recognized by special tests.

If only part of your penis fails to get hard, or doesn't get as hard as the rest, or if when your penis enlarges it hurts or bends in a way that it did not previously, there is likely to be a physical problem in your penis and you should see your doctor. He will probably send you to a specialist urologist.

Should your penis seem to be habitually smaller than previously, feel cold, or appear to have changed in colour, you should seek medical advice, because these changes are often signs of penile blood flow problems.

If you have pain in or swelling of a testicle, or an obvious change in your waterworks (needing to go frequently, burning or scalding, passing much more urine than usual, difficulty urinating, and so on) see your doctor without delay. If there is any discomfort when you ejaculate, blood in your semen or difficulty ejaculating normally, these must be checked out medically.

If you feel generally unwell or run down, if you have lost weight without dieting, or have pain or lumps for which you do not already have a precise medical diagnosis, you need to be examined.

If you have noticed changes in your vision, sense of smell, or hearing, or if you are aware of some loss of normal feeling or sensation, or of any weakness or clumsiness of the muscles in any part of your body, these must be medically assessed. Any unusual turns, headaches, or change in your speech should also be investigated.

Should you decide not to seek a general medical examination first-up, because you feel well physically, and have no symptoms other than impotence, you are probably not running much of a risk that some serious medical complaint is being missed. If, however, your erection problem fails to respond to the careful application of the self-help procedures to be described, I would **strongly** urge you to have a thorough general physical examination, **even if** you think you are perfectly healthy!

It is a medical myth that normal early morning erections, or normal erections during the night, mean that no physical factors could be involved in your impotence, although some doctors are not aware of this. It is also untrue that if you can get a normal erection in one situation (masturbation or with a particular partner), but not another, then there can be nothing wrong physically! Even many doctors are unaware of this second medical myth, as it has only been found to be untrue in quite recent times. It is a fact, that if you have completely normal erections in some situation (when you wake up, during sleep, or in some form of sexual activity), this excludes quite a number of possible physical disease contributions to impotence, but **not all!** For example, important penile blood flow problems, both in arteries and veins, can exist, even though you get a normal erection under certain circumstances.

Remember that **your partner's genital structure may be compounding your erectile problem!** If her vagina is very loose and slack, she may not be able to give you enough stimulation after penetration, contributing to your loss of erection. If her vagina is too tight, it may be difficult to penetrate her, unless you have a very firm erection. You may also lose your erection while fumbling around trying to get it in. If either of these possibilities could apply in your case, **gently** talk them over with your partner. **Under no circumstances give her any grounds for thinking that you are blaming her for your problem, or complaining, or putting her down!** Remember that at worst, any vaginal problem can only be one factor contributing to your difficulty, not the whole cause!

The guiding principles in evaluating yourself for possible physical contributions to impotence, must be crystal clear to you. They are:

1. Ideally, you would have a full general physical examination.
2. If you have any physical symptoms or abnormalities, particularly the ones detailed above, see your doctor. If you need to consult him about these, you might as well also ask him to give you a thorough general physical examination.
3. If you feel completely well, and have no symptoms other than impotence, you will probably come to no harm if you choose not to have a general physical examination first-up. However, **if your impotence does not respond to the measures outlined in this book, you should then have a full physical examination, no matter how well you feel!**

Always remember the other side of the medical situation — a normal general physical examination, and the complete absence of physical symptoms, do not in any way guarantee that there are no physical factors contributing to your impotence!

Psychological Contributions

For convenience, these have been divided into personal and relationship issues.

Personal Factors

It is vitally important to check out the possibility that you have what is technically known as a 'depressive illness', which is a very common ailment. This is quite a complex issue medically, especially since you can have this without really feeling depressed. If you **often** feel down, gloomy, guilty, don't like yourself, wonder whether life is really worth living, don't sleep very well, have little interest in things that previously you enjoyed, find that you have to really push yourself to perform many ordinary tasks, feel tense, anxious, irritable, don't really enjoy your food as you did previously, lack energy, or get tired very easily, have lost weight, can't concentrate or find your memory is not good, then you may very well have a depressive illness. Of course, nobody with this disorder has **all** these complaints! If you have some of them, **even if you don't feel particularly depressed, check it out with a doctor!** Having a depressive illness is actually good news, because often it is relatively easy to treat, and when you are over it, your potency may be restored without doing anything else.

Check whether you are often anxious and tense, or feeling stressed. If so, see if you can work out why, and what you can do to overcome whatever things are making you like that. Even if you can't find or change the causes, you can often greatly reduce your anxiety and tension by the regular practice of a formal relaxation technique, such as the ones described in appendix 5.

It is worth knowing that **caffeine** (the stimulant drug in coffee, tea and cola beverages), often **makes some people anxious and tense!** If you drink these, and feel they could be affecting you, experiment to see whether stopping them **completely,** makes you feel any better. If you try this, it may take a few months off all caffeine before you can decide if it is relevant, and you may feel miserable for about a week, because of caffeine withdrawal effects.

If you often feel nervous or anxious, and drink alcohol nearly every day, or to excess, this may be contributing to the way you feel, even though the immediate effect of alcohol is to temporarily reduce anxiety. **If this is a possibility, stop drinking completely for a month and see how you feel!** Remember my comments about difficulty stopping drinking, mentioned earlier.

It is very important to know whether or not you feel anxious when you are in sexual situations, since there is little chance that you will then erect adequately. This is true, regardless of the cause of your anxiety, but especially relevant if you are worried about your sexual performance. Try to work out what actual thoughts you have running through your mind, when you are making love. Are you thinking about how well or otherwise you will perform? Are you thinking about how your partner will react if you don't deliver the goods? Is your mind on any other unhelpful factors? If you are not sure, close your eyes and run through in detail, in your mind, a recent sexual encounter, paying attention to your thoughts and feelings. **If you felt anxious, you were probably thinking anxiety-making thoughts!** What were they? Write down the kinds of unhelpful thoughts you typically have in sexual situations. You will use this information in working out exactly what remedial exercises you have to do (chapter 11).

Check to see whether feelings of anger, guilt, shame, unhappiness, disgust or jealousy could possibly be relevant to your sexual performance, directly or indirectly exerting an adverse effect upon it. Are any such emotions interfering with your conditions for being sexually responsive?

Check to see whether you work at **actively trying to make an erection occur,** when you want one. If you are, this destructive habit must cease forever, since the more you try, the more difficult it will be to get a hard-on. **Erections cannot be made to occur, they can only be allowed to occur!** Don't get into a war with your penis, trying to force it to stand up — it will win every time!

If you have been using this book as suggested, taking it a chapter at a time, and doing everything I have asked, you will already have a written list of the main sexual myths that handicap you in your quest for sexual happiness, and a second list of these, rewritten in logical, rational terms. You will also have a written, detailed summary of your conditions for being sexually responsive. If you haven't got these, **don't move on under any circumstances** until you have re-read the relevant chapters, and thoroughly done the exercises described. Make sure you read your final lists of logical, rational sexual beliefs, and of your conditions, with feeling, each and every day!

Relationship Factors

Let me warn you in advance, that it is very difficult to self-evaluate objectively and accurately for relationship contributions to your impotence. That should not stop you trying, preferably with the help of your partner, but do not be surprised if you don't get very far.

Remember my rules of thumb:

1. Your partner's responses to your sexual problems often, if not usually, inadvertently make them worse, even in the very best relationships.
2. Your prospects for overcoming your impotence with your partner, hinge on the **true quality** of your relationship with her.

Check out the following possibilities, being as truthful as you can:

1. Have you **honestly** and **thoroughly** discussed your impotence, **and your rational and irrational concerns about it,** with your partner? Do you really know in detail, exactly how she feels about it? If not, what has made it difficult to do so? How can you get around this deficient communication?
2. In your lovemaking, have you been able to let her know **exactly** what kind of stimulation you wish and need? If not, what has made this difficult or embarrassing for you, and what can you do about it? If you have, but are still not getting it, then why not?
3. In your lovemaking, have you **both** modified your erotic techniques and expectations, to compensate for the changes age has made to your erection process? If you are not **absolutely certain** what these changes are, re-read chapter 4.
4. During lovemaking, do you tend to accept, or be left with, responsibility for her arousal and response? Is she inappropriately passive? Is she really interested and involved? What can you do about these issues?

5. Have you both inadvertently allowed lovemaking to become something of a routine, so that it is no longer very exciting or arousing? What does your partner think about this possibility? If it has happened, what can you both do about it?

6. Are **any** of her responses to your erectile difficulty aggravating it? Carefully re-read chapters 8 and 9, with this question in mind, remembering that **even loving, well-meaning responses can sometimes inadvertently aggravate impotence!**

7. Are you resentful or disappointed about some aspects of your partner's non-sexual behaviour? Are there things she does or does not do that displease you? What about her feelings about your behaviour? Are these non-sexual issues possibly having an unhelpful effect on your sexual relationship? If so, what can you do to overcome them? Can you both communicate openly, honestly and comfortably about your dissatisfactions?

If it is clear that there are problems in your general relationship, related to or affecting your sexual functioning, these will have to be talked over and sorted out **before** you make any formal attempt to solve your erection problem. Provided you both can sit down and talk **constructively** about difficulties, you may be able to overcome them yourselves. If you can't frankly discuss your problems together, without arguing or getting upset, or because it is too hurtful, you would be very well advised to together consult a professional marriage counsellor. Remember, **there is very little prospect of you again being potent with your partner, while there are significant problems between you!** Relationship difficulties **must** be overcome, **before** you attempt to directly tackle your sexual problem!

Preparing for Direct Treatment of Your Impotence

It is important to start the direct attack on your erection problem with as much going for you as possible. With this philosophy in mind, **before you move on to the exercises specifically directed at regaining your potency,** first attend to the following:

1. Work at giving up smoking. Get assistance if necessary.
2. Do what you can about any drug or chemical factors which may be contributing to your impotence.

3. If you drink alcohol or caffeine, see if they are aggravating your problem.
4. If indicated, check out with your doctor any possible physical contributions to your erectile difficulty, and get any necessary medical treatment.
5. If your partner's genital structure is contributing to your difficulties, discuss this with her, and take appropriate remedial action (pelvic muscle exercise if vagina too loose, gynaecological advice if vagina too tight).
6. If you could have a depressive illness, seek medical advice and treatment.
7. Minimize any stresses, and work to overcome the adverse effects of stress, by regular formal relaxation (appendix 5).
8. Deal with frequent anxiety and tension by overcoming any reversible causes, and by regular formal relaxation.
9. Deal with any significant relationship problems.
10. If anger, guilt, shame, unhappiness, disgust or jealousy appear relevant, see what you can do to overcome them. Thoroughly discuss these issues with your partner, and perhaps also consider using thought stopping (appendix 3), relaxation (appendix 5), desensitization (appendix 8), the Premack principle (appendix 2), or autosuggestion (appendix 9), to reduce or overcome their impact.

The management of anxiety related to the sexual situation will be discussed in the next chapter.

Chapter 11

WHAT YOU CAN NOW DO TO HELP YOURSELF

The process of overcoming your erection problem and regaining your confidence in your erectile capacity, revolves around homework exercises and a number of interlocking 'requirements'. The more of these requirements that can be properly met, the better your outlook for success. They will first be listed, then discussed.

Requirement 1
You must accept the fact that it will probably take some considerable time to overcome your problem!

Requirement 2
If you have a partner you must communicate about your problem openly and honestly!

Requirement 3
You must practise what is required regularly, thoroughly and under reasonably good conditions!

Requirement 4
You must develop the correct mental attitude to sexual expression!

Requirement 5
You must 'take the pressure off your penis'!

Requirement 6
You must become personally involved in sex only when you are genuinely sexually aroused and interested!

Requirement 7
You must make sure that your conditions for being sexually responsive are adequately met!

Requirement 8
You must make sure you get adequate stimulation!

Requirement 9
You must focus mentally on the stimulation you are receiving during sexual contact!

Obviously, some of these 'requirements' overlap, and they are certainly not listed in the order in which they must be met.

Requirements 6 and 7 have been discussed in chapter 6. By now, you will have a crystal clear idea of your own personal conditions for being sexually responsive. You will never again make the unbelievably stupid mistake of getting into a sexual situation, in which there is any expectation by either yourself or your partner, that you will be sexually responsive, unless your conditions for being responsive are reasonably met! This of course does not necessarily mean that you will avoid all sexual contact when your conditions are inadequately met! You might then feel like and enjoy naked cuddling and fondling, or manipulating your partner to orgasm, without wanting or expecting to become aroused yourself.

How Long Will it Take to Overcome Your Problem?

This will of course depend on many factors. The important rules are:
1. Make haste slowly!
2. Go at your own comfortable pace!
3. Do **not** move from one step to the next, until you have **thoroughly** mastered the present one!

Under good conditions, where everything goes more or less according to plan, it will probably take you at least 3 months to master what needs to be done. It may take much longer, largely depending on how much time you have available to practise. You can't **make** your problem disappear, you can only **allow** it to go away! It is better to move along slowly and steadily, and get there in the end, than to rush and perhaps miss out on success!

After your actual erectile performance has been restored, so that you are again having normal intercourse, it will take **many additional months,** before you are once again truly confident of your erectile ability, and no longer have occasional thoughts about whether or not you will erect adequately!

What About Open and Honest Communication With Your Partner?

A truly caring and cooperative partner is **your greatest asset** in overcoming your problem! However, if she is to help you maximally, she must understand as much as possible about your problem, and **especially,** how you feel about it! Let her know just how being impotent makes you feel, even if it sounds over-dramatic! You will certainly find that sharing with her your anxieties, shame, guilt, anger, and so on will make you feel much better, and take a lot of psychological pressure off your shoulders, and even more importantly, off your penis!

How to Get the Most from What You Have to Practise

You will find there are a variety of exercises for you to master and perform. As a general rule, a little done frequently tends to be more effective than a large amount done occasionally. Try to arrange your daily/weekly schedule so that you can spend on average 30 to 60 minutes of **prime time** each day, working at various aspects of what has to be done. Prime time means when you are alert, able to concentrate fully, and feeling reasonably good. By and large, it is a waste of time to try to force yourself to practise your exercises under poor conditions, for example, when you are in a hurry, uptight, tired and so on. You may have to have a long hard look at your routine and your priorities, to permit the necessary practice under really good conditions, and **you will probably have to ruthlessly prune off**

a few non-essential activities or chores! However, **if you really wish to succeed,** you will **somehow** find enough regular prime time, **whatever the difficulties** that have to be overcome to achieve this! All exercises must be performed **exactly** as described and **very thoroughly!**

What is the Correct Mental Attitude to Sexual Expression?

Lovemaking means literally that—making love with someone you care about, giving and receiving pleasure, both physical and psychological. **An erect penis and intercourse are not in any way necessary for it, and it doesn't always have to result in orgasm!**

As thus defined, lovemaking can **never** be a failure! Whatever happens, it can only be a success!

Having this attitude is one of the most important requirements for overcoming your erection problem! A variety of effective methods for changing your faulty attitudes to this desirable one are described in appendix 1, should you need to do more work on them.

How Do You Take the Pressure Off Your Penis?

Make an absolute commitment, to yourself, and with your partner, that **under no circumstances will vaginal penetration be attempted during lovemaking, until you have completely and thoroughly worked through your entire corrective exercise programme!** This of course does not in any way mean that you can't make love! **You can do that any time you wish!** However, when you do, even if you happen to have a perfect erection, under no circumstances are you to attempt vaginal penetration! Use non-intercourse methods for bringing each other to orgasm, should you individually or both wish to climax on a particular occasion.

You ignore this rule at your own grave peril! It is designed to take all performance pressure out of the lovemaking situation, so that you can again begin to relate sexually, without the dreadful spectre of 'failure' (meaning not having an erection adequate for vaginal penetration) wrecking your mutual pleasure, and steadily making your problem of impotence much worse. When vaginal penetration is not a lovemaking option, **whether or not you erect becomes completely irrelevant,** since the only function of an erection is to enable penetration.

You know, of course, that you do not have to have an erection, in order to be able to be manipulated to orgasm. Unless there is a drug or a physical disorder affecting your ejaculation mechanism, you can climax and ejaculate without an erection. If you have any difficulties achieving this, follow the detailed suggestions in the next chapter.

How to Make Sure You Get Adequate Stimulation

The only way you can be certain that you will get adequate **physical** stimulation, is to instruct your partner exactly how you wish your genital area to be manipulated. Even if she knows you very well, your exact needs will vary from occasion to occasion, and she simply can't read your mind! Remember, it is **your** responsibility to make sure that you get the kind of stimulation you want or need, where you want it, for as long as you want it.

You will get adequate **mental** stimulation only if most of your conditions for being sexually responsive are met — see chapter 6. It may help to enhance your mental stimulation during lovemaking, if you tune in to a fantasy that appeals to you. Exactly how to get the maximum benefit from this approach is described in detail in appendix 7.

Why it is Important to Focus Mentally on the Stimulation You are Receiving During Sexual Contact

The **key** to getting the maximum arousal and sexual excitement from adequate physical stimulation, is your ability to focus on the **physical sensations** you are experiencing at any one moment, whether they result from your partner touching you, or you touching her. This is a skill which requires practice, and you will be shown how to master it in appendix 4.

The Sequence of Events for Now Tackling Your Erection Problem

I am assuming that by now, you have evaluated for physical and chemical factors possibly contributing to your impotence, and for a depressive illness, and already taken any appropriate action. These issues, and the others summarized at the end of the last chapter, **must** be attended to **before** you begin working directly on your problem!

Remember particularly, if you feel that there are significant problems in your relationship with your partner, which interfere with your ability to communicate freely and be comfortable and close together, you **must** overcome them **before** directly tackling the erection problem — see chapter 10.

If you have a partner, make sure you have thoroughly discussed your problem, and exactly how you feel about it, with her. Remember, the overwhelming majority of women who in any way care about you as a person, will be supportive, understanding, and helpful. Explain the absolutely crucial importance of taking the pressure off your penis, and discuss with her how this can be achieved, as described earlier in this chapter. Contract with her that **under no circumstances** will vaginal penetration ever be attempted during lovemaking, until you have completely finished the formal exercise programme. Point out to her the **positive** aspects of an enforced period of lovemaking without the option of intercourse! It will compel you both to smarten up your non-intercourse lovemaking techniques, and perhaps inspire you both to try out a range of new, potentially more enjoyable, stimulative manoeuvres.

Next, check to make sure you have **thoroughly** done the exercises described in chapters 5 and 6 — **these are absolutely essential before you move on any further!** If having done these, you still don't feel very confident that you **really** believe and are committed to the attitude that lovemaking can be truly great, even without an erection, what do you do? Tackle **now** the specific exercises directed at attaining this key attitude, described in appendix 1. Be **absolutely certain** that you get this attitude right **before** you move on!

Now work out, and write down, the approximate times each day, when you are going to practise your exercises. Remember, you need prime time, and if you are really motivated to succeed, you will somehow find the time, whatever the practical difficulties!

Next, select those individual preliminary exercises from the list below, which are either essential or seem relevant to your particular situation. If in doubt as to whether or not you need to do a particular exercise, **do it anyway!** It is better to play safe and have as much going for you as possible! As a general rule, **only** when you have **fully mastered** these **individual** exercises, do you begin the **joint** exercises with your partner. The practical details of these various procedures are described for convenience in the appendix.

Individual Exercises

1. Thought Stopping

If you tend to have unhelpful thoughts in your mind in the sexual situation, especially any thoughts about how you will perform, master this as a way of getting rid of them.

2. Sensuality Training

You should always do these exercises.

3. Self-Relaxation

If you are anxious or tense in the sexual situation, or in anticipation of it, master deliberate relaxation, so that you can use it as a way of getting rid of this very destructive anxiety and tension. If you feel that life generally is stressful, use regular, deliberate, formal relaxation as a way of reducing the harmful effects of this stress.

4. Pelvic Muscle Exercise

You should do this, no matter what.

5. Fantasy Training

You should always do this.

6. Desensitization

If in spite of the use of thought stopping and relaxation, you are still **in any way** nervous or anxious in the sexual situation, or in anticipation of it, you should use this procedure.

7. Autosuggestion

This is designed to help alter unhelpful sexual attitudes, based on myths. Use it, if you feel you are still adversely affected by these!

8. Individual Erectile Exercises

These are absolutely essential in all cases, but should **not be attempted until all the other relevant individual exercises have been thoroughly mastered.**

Joint Exercises

Do not attempt these until you have **fully** mastered **all** your relevant individual exercises!

There are 3 things to do, and they are **all** important!

1. Sexual Communication Exercise

Do this every day, as described in appendix 11.

2. Shared Sensuality Exercises

You can begin these as soon as you have finished your individual exercises. You do **not** have to wait until you have completed the sexual communication exercise! The goals of the first step must be **thoroughly** achieved before the second step is commenced.

3. Joint Erectile Exercises

These must **not** be attempted until **both** parts of the shared sensuality exercise have been performed, and their goals **fully** achieved!

Remember to make haste slowly with all the exercises!

Obviously, if you do not have a partner with whom you can perform the shared exercises, these cannot be done. While this makes your task more difficult, **it certainly does not mean that you can't overcome your problem!** In this situation, put all your efforts into the individual exercises, and **really make them count!** Also, carefully study and think about the suggestions for lovemaking with a new partner — see chapter 12 and appendix 16.

If you have a steady partner, but she won't cooperate in the treatment programme, you have relationship problems, or, she has her own sexual difficulties, and these issues should be dealt with as best possible, perhaps with the assistance of a professional.

What to do Now

1. Study the Schematic Overview of the Progressive Self-Help Programme, beginning on the next page. Make sure you understand what you are supposed to have already done, and what you have yet to do.
2. **Then,** read chapter 12.
3. **Then,** begin practising and mastering your individual exercises.
4. **Then,** should you have a partner, begin practising and mastering your joint exercises.

SCHEMATIC OVERVIEW OF THE PROGRESSIVE SELF-HELP PROGRAMME DESCRIBED IN THIS BOOK

Record Each Day's Work in a Notebook!

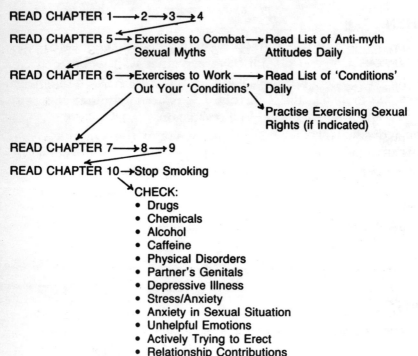

READ CHAPTER 1⟶2⟶3⟶4

READ CHAPTER 5⟶Exercises to Combat⟶Read List of Anti-myth
                    Sexual Myths   Attitudes Daily

READ CHAPTER 6⟶Exercises to Work⟶Read List of 'Conditions'
                    Out Your 'Conditions'   Daily

                                        Practise Exercising Sexual
                                        Rights (if indicated)

READ CHAPTER 7⟶8⟶9

READ CHAPTER 10⟶Stop Smoking

                    CHECK:
                    • Drugs
                    • Chemicals
                    • Alcohol
                    • Caffeine
                    • Physical Disorders
                    • Partner's Genitals
                    • Depressive Illness
                    • Stress/Anxiety
                    • Anxiety in Sexual Situation
                    • Unhelpful Emotions
                    • Actively Trying to Erect
                    • Relationship Contributions

> NOW TAKE APPROPRIATE REMEDIAL ACTION
> BEFORE DIRECTLY TACKLING IMPOTENCE

THEN:

READ CHAPTER 11⟶Thoroughly Discuss Problem with Your Partner
                    (if not previously done).
                    ↓
                    Contract to Take Pressure off the Penis in
                    Lovemaking
                    ↓
                    Assess Belief in the Key Sexual Attitude
                    IF NOT CONFIDENT, DO EXERCISES IN
                    APPENDIX 1, NOW
                    ↓
                    Work Out When You Can Practise Your
                    Exercises Each Day
                    ↓
                    Select Individual Exercises

THEN:

READ CHAPTER 12

THEN:

1. PRACTISE THE INDICATED INDIVIDUAL EXERCISES FROM THE APPENDIX

   When Fully Mastered ──────▶ Practise Individual Erectile Exercise, Step 4, at Least Twice Weekly, Until You Begin the Joint Erectile Exercises.

2. PRACTISE THE JOINT EXERCISES IF YOU HAVE A COOPERATIVE PARTNER

   Shared Sensuality
   Exercise, Step 1,   PLUS Sexual Communication Exercise

   Shared Sensuality
   Exercise, Step 2,   PLUS Sexual Communication Exercise

   Joint Erectile
   Exercises,   PLUS Sexual Communication Exercise

OUTCOME

1. SUCCESSFUL TREATMENT ──────▶ Resume Intercourse in Lovemaking, but Following Special Post-Treatment Hints (Appendix 14).

   If No Partner, Additionally Follow Hints in Chapter 12 and Appendices 10 and 16.

2. UNSUCCESSFUL TREATMENT ──▶ Medical Investigation and any Needed Treatment

   Expert Sex Therapy

   • SUCCESS ──▶ Resume Intercourse, Following Post-Treatment Hints/No-Partner Hints

   • FAILURE ──▶ Second Opinion

   Check Options (Chapter 12)

   Decision on Options

Chapter 12

SPECIAL ISSUES

The Role of Specialists in Treating Impotence

The Endocrinologist
This physician specializes in diseases of endocrine glands — the body structures which produce hormones. The endocrinologist is expert in diagnosing and treating hormonal disorders, but has had no special training in the overall management of sexual problems. Treatments mostly involve the use of drugs aimed at overcoming hormone problems.

The Neurologist
This physician specializes in diseases of the brain, spinal cord, nerves and muscles. The neurologist has had special training in the diagnosis and management of these problems, but not in the treatment of sexual disorders. When there is a treatment available for a neurological disorder, it usually involves drugs, or in some cases, surgery.

The Psychiatrist
This physician is concerned with the psychological aspects of medicine, and may or may not have had special training and experience in the management of sexual problems. The contribution of a psychiatrist who has such training lies in helping overcome the psychological factors contributing to or maintaining a sexual difficulty. Psychiatrists also have expertise in helping couples cope with marital or relationship problems. Before consulting with a

psychiatrist about a problem of impotence, check with your family doctor or the psychiatrist's secretary, to make sure that psychiatrist deals with sexual problems, as not all do.

The Psychologist

This professional is not medically qualified and has had therefore no training in the various physical disorders and chemical agents which may contribute to an erection problem. Clinical psychologists, like psychiatrists, may have special expertise in the management of the psychological issues relevant to a case of impotence. Before consulting with one, check to make sure that psychologist has had training and experience in the management of sexual problems, as not all have.

The Sex Therapist

Individuals who practise as sex therapists specialize in the management of sexual problems. They may or may not be medically qualified — some are by basic training, clinical psychologists. Medically qualified sex therapists come from many specialties — some were family physicians, some psychiatrists, some gynaecologists, and so on. Their training and experience in the sexual field is more important than their original specialty.

The Urologist

This specialist is a surgeon concerned with disorders of the male genitals and the urinary system — kidneys and bladder — of both sexes. The urologist has special skill in diagnosing and treating disorders of these structures. Few have had special training in the treatment of impotence other than by hormones and surgery.

The Vascular Surgeon

This specialist is concerned with the diagnosis and treatment of disorders of blood vessels, both arteries and veins. The vascular surgeon has very important skills in diagnosing vascular contributions to impotence, which are now known to be extremely common, and may be able to correct certain blood flow problems surgically. However, vascular surgeons have had no special training in the overall treatment of sexual problems.

Some Special Investigations which May be Used in Diagnosing the Causes of Impotence

Nocturnal Penile Tumescence Monitoring (NPT test)

Abnormalities of penile erection during sleep (see chapter 3) may give information as to the presence of physical disorders contributing to an erectile problem. This investigation can be done in a variety of different ways, each with its own advantages and disadvantages. It gives no information as to the precise nature of any physical disorders contributing to impotence. Sometimes there are considerable technical difficulties in interpreting what the test result means, and it is not absolutely reliable in detecting physical disorders. At best, it is a screening test for many physical abnormalities.

Penile Arterial Blood Flow Measurement

With the growing realization that abnormalities of the flow of blood into the penis are very common in impotent men, this measurement has become increasingly important. There are several ways of doing it, some more accurate than others. If the test result is abnormal, it gives no information as to where the blockage to blood flow is located — it could be in the abdomen, in the pelvis, in the arteries of the penis or in several or all of these locations. The test gives no information about the condition of the very small arteries in the penis, so that a normal result does **not** rule out the possibility of blockages in these very small arteries, which may in fact be quite common.

Arteriography

This is a special x-ray technique for locating the site or sites of blockages to arteries, and abnormal connections between arteries and veins. A special chemical which can be seen on an x-ray is injected into a large artery, enabling the flow of blood along the branches of that artery to be seen. A general or a spinal anaesthetic is necessary for arteriography of the blood supply to the penis.

Cavernosography

This is a special x-ray technique showing the flow of blood through the pressure cylinders of the penis, and its pattern of exit through the draining veins. The procedure is similar to arteriography but the chemical is injected directly into the penis using only a local anaesthetic.

The Role of Drugs in the Treatment of Impotence

Testosterone (Male Hormone)

Many impotent men are given testosterone, either in tablet form or by injection, when they consult a doctor. Unless you have been proven to suffer from testosterone deficiency (a blood test is required), this amounts to a shot in the dark. There is no doubt in my mind, based on experience, that **some** men who do **not** suffer from testosterone deficiency benefit, although certainly **most do not!** If this treatment helps when you are not testosterone deficient, it may do so by exerting a strong 'placebo' effect — a purely psychological benefit based on your hope and expectation that it will help! Some men who really don't need extra testosterone, find that the drug greatly (but temporarily) increases their sexual desire. They may become so sexually excited, that this helps them to overcome the effects of anxiety about performance, which previously was blocking their ability to erect. A few successful sexual experiences thus achieved may restore such a man's sexual confidence to the extent that no further hormone supplements or other treatments are needed. It is to be emphasized strongly however, that a beneficial response to extra testosterone which is really **not** needed by the body, is unusual — mostly the drug has no useful effect at all! Sometimes, unnecessary extra testosterone makes the impotent man's plight **worse,** by artificially increasing his sexual drive, so that he becomes even more frustrated by his inability to erect adequately!

If a doctor suggests giving you testosterone as a treatment for impotence, I would urge you to decline, until a proper blood test has been carried out to determine whether or not you are in fact deficient in testosterone. If you are, then further investigations often have to be conducted to find out the cause of the problem, before the diagnostic situation is confused by the administration of male hormone.

Synthetic Testosterone-like Drugs

The same comments apply here as with testosterone itself. In general, they are often less satisfactory than testosterone, should you genuinely need male hormone replacement.

Other Hormone Treatments

If your impotence is due to or associated with other hormone disorders, these will usually need some form of specific drug treatment. However, such treatments can have no beneficial effects on potency, unless you suffer from the disorder they are designed to treat!

Blood Vessel Dilating Drugs

If blockage of the flow of blood into the penis is a factor contributing to your impotence, then drugs which might enlarge (dilate) the arteries to the penis could be worth a try. However, they are **very rarely effective** in improving potency!

Minor Tranquillizers

These are drugs like diazepam (Valium). They combat anxiety, and are **occasionally** helpful in reducing it to a degree sufficient to enable predominantly anxiety-based impotence to be overcome. **More usually, they are totally unhelpful!**

Antidepressants

These may improve erectile potency if the problem is associated with a depressive illness.

Other Drugs for Impotence

Human ingenuity has responded to the desperation of impotent men over the centuries by devising all types of chemical treatments, none of which are consistently effective, and some of which are frankly dangerous, for example, Spanish fly. Because of the placebo response, which remember, is a purely psychological effect, some of these preparations may help some men, at least temporarily. However, the same benefit would have been achieved if these men had been given a tablet consisting of pure sugar, provided they had been strongly led to believe that it would help them!

As medical science progresses, it is quite likely that drugs which can specifically benefit potency in at least some cases of impotence will ultimately be developed. Until that happy day arrives, don't waste your money on useless drug remedies!

Injection Treatment for Impotence

A lot is now being written about injection treatment for impotence which is becoming available in various centres around the country. The method involves injecting drugs directly into the erectile tissue of the penis. The drugs most commonly used are papaverine and phentolamine. Normally, erection occurs soon after the injection and lasts from a few minutes to many hours depending on the dose of drugs used.

Sometimes, obtaining an erection by this means and using it to have intercourse with gives the man confidence and allays his fear of failure so that just one injection is required. Other men require an injection whenever they want to have an erection. Patients and their partners are now being taught how to carry out the injections themselves so that they can use this method of obtaining erections at home when they want to have intercourse. However, this form of treatment does not work in every case of impotence and it is not without risk. We do not know what the long term consequences of repeated injections will be. Sometimes, if the dose of the drug is too large the erection lasts too long and requires treatment (often an injection into the penis of a different drug) to make it go down.

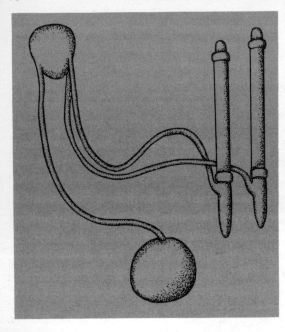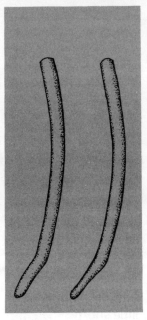

Fig. 5 (Left) An inflatable penile prosthesis
Fig. 6 (Right) A semi-rigid penile prosthesis

Surgical Treatments for Impotence

When impotence is largely the result of blood flow problems to, within, or from the penis, in some cases vascular surgical procedures can restore potency. A vascular surgeon is the appropriate specialist to advise you about this possibility.

When impotence of any cause, be it largely psychological, or mainly due to physical problems, proves incurable in spite of properly conducted treatment, a man has 2 options. He may choose to accept the difficulty, and concentrate on making the most of sexual relating without the option of intercourse with an erect penis. Alternatively, he may decide to have a penile implant or prosthesis inserted.

There are basically two types of implants. The first is a truly ingenious inflatable device. Pump-up cylinders made of inert material are surgically implanted into each of the 2 pressure cylinders. They are connected by fine tubing to a fluid reservoir implanted inside the abdominal wall, and a pump located in the scrotum (the bag of skin containing the testicles). When an erection is desired, the man pumps fluid into the penile cylinders until he has the required degree of erection. When he no longer has any use for his erection, he deflates his penis, using the pump in his scrotum. This device is shown in figure 5.

These devices work well, but are extremely expensive and have some technical disadvantages. For example, the connecting tubes sometimes block and further surgery is required to repair them. As with any major surgery there are possible complications, such as infection and the possible hazards of anaesthesia.

The second type of prosthesis consists of 2 inert, flexible rods (figure 6) which are surgically implanted into each of the 2 pressure cylinders of the penis. These rods largely fill the space inside the pressure cylinders, so that at all times the man has an erect penis adequate for penetration. His penis will be firm but not hard, and it will remain pointed in whatever position it is placed. It will be a little shorter than his previous maximum erectile size, and there will be some decrease in the maximum thickness of the penis, because it would not be comfortable to use rods which completely filled the pressure cylinders. The surgery to insert these rods is relatively simple, and certainly much less difficult than with the inflatable device. The rods, however, have technical disadvantages in certain cases.

Any man contemplating implant surgery, must fully understand the following essential facts.

1. The insertion of either of these devices **permanently** destroys the ability to get a natural erection because erectile tissue is destroyed. The penis will therefore not erect over and above the penile size produced by the implant.

2. All that surgery achieves is the ability to penetrate one's partner! It makes **no difference** to sexual interest, sexual pleasure, ejaculation or orgasm!

3. If one has a partner, she **must** be involved in the decision making about this type of surgery. Unless she is in **full** agreement with the procedure when it has been thoroughly explained to her, **do not** have the operation! For example, some women really have no interest in further sexual contact, and after a period without sex, may find intercourse actively

unpleasant! All the surgery then achieves is an increase in unhappiness and frustration for both partners, although the man's penis may look great in the locker room at the golf-club!

4. When **both** partners **genuinely** desire intercourse, and find lovemaking without it less than fully satisfying, implant surgery leads to excellent results.

5. A urologist experienced in the use of both types of implant is in the best position to decide what type of prosthesis would be most suitable for you, bearing in mind a variety of technical considerations. Let him advise you!

Other Treatments

Penile Volume Biofeedback Therapy

Biofeedback means giving an individual immediate information about the present state of some body organ or function. For example, if you were connected to a machine that made a beeping sound each time your heart beats, you would be getting biofeedback about your heart rate. Extraordinary as it may seem, many humans who are motivated enough to put in the necessary practice with a biofeedback machine, can learn a useful degree of voluntary control over the body function concerned. One can, for example, learn to voluntarily control heart rate, blood pressure, skin temperature and so on. Using complex electronic instruments, many men can learn a useful degree of voluntary control over the size of their penis. Occasionally this approach has been helpful in impotence, particularly when psychological factors have been largely responsible for it. Few therapists possess the necessary instrumentation, and the technique is rarely used.

Acupuncture

I have seen patients who have reported improvement in their erectile capacity, even back to normal, after acupuncture treatment. I have no idea how this would work, but perhaps, at least in some cases, it is a placebo reaction — due to a psychological response of hope and expectation that a particular treatment will work. Most of my patients who have tried acupuncture for their impotence have reported no benefit. However, apart from disappointment, it can do you no harm, as long as it is competently performed.

External Penile Splints

There are various types. One variety attach around the penis, acting like a mechanical splint to a broken leg, providing enough rigidity for penetration. Most men report that they are neither particularly effective nor comfortable. A second type consists of a hollow, firm, artificial penis (dildo) which fits completely over your non-erect penis. There is no difficulty penetrating your partner, but the necessary thickness of the gadget gives you no real feeling of being inside a vagina. In a sense, you are having intercourse with the device, while it is having intercourse with your partner! Some men find that the relief of anxiety about getting hard enough to penetrate their partner, actually enables them to begin to erect naturally in the sexual situation. Most men find these hollow devices unsatisfactory, but some swear by them!

Correctaid

This in many ways looks like a condom but it has the advantage of actually inducing an erection. It has been described as a tumescence (erection) assistance device. It consists of a transparent silicone rubber cylinder incorporating a silicone tube. The flaccid penis is placed inside the device in which a vacuum is then created by suction on the adjoining tube. The negative pressure inside the device induces penile erection which lasts until the device is removed.

The device is used during intercourse and many women say that it feels very little different from a normally erect penis covered with a contraceptive sheath. When first seen, the device may be a little off-putting to some men and their partners but experience shows that very few couples are unable to accept it and that it is a useful aid to the management of impotence.

As the device is matched to the size of the man's penis, he has to supply details of the length and diameter of his penis to the distributor* who then supplies an appropriately-sized device.

Hypnosis

Hypnosis is essentially a state where you are relaxed, focused mentally on what is being said, and very susceptible to appropriate suggestions. You can induce a state of hypnosis by yourself, or with the assistance of a therapist. There are many different ways in which the hypnotic state can be used to assist impotent men, and whatever approach is used by a skilled therapist, will be **individually tailored** to the specific needs of a particular man. Hypnosis is merely one of a variety of psychological treatments which can be used in impotence, and it is most often used in conjunction with other methods, rather than by itself.

Things to Avoid

These fall into 2 categories — those to be avoided because they are useless, but harmless, and those which may actually cause harm.

Most drugs or preparations which can be legitimately purchased without a prescription from a doctor, are harmless but useless. Avoid illicit or street drugs. You never know exactly what you are buying, and no drug exists which will effectively overcome impotence! You may also find yourself in serious trouble with the law. This is true even for marijuana which in some circles has an undeserved reputation for improving sexual performance, and an equally undeserved reputation for being harmless and perfectly safe! Remember what has been said about the placebo effect of any drug — if you strongly believe that it will help, it may very well do so, if your problem is largely psychological. However, the existence of a significant placebo effect with any drug is **not** in any way a justification for its use!

The main treatments to be very careful about are devices or gadgets which in any way fit tightly around or constrict the penis. These may

*Genesis Medical Limited, Freepost 24, London W1

on occasions cause serious damage. Anything which interferes with blood flowing out of the penis may lead to blood clotting in the penis, which is not only very painful, but can lead to **irreversible damage** to the normal erection mechanism! If you feel tempted to try any such gadgets, first consult with a urologist or vascular surgeon, and show them to him!

The Special Problems of Impotent Men Without a Partner

It is usually much easier to overcome a problem of impotence if you have a cooperative partner with whom you can thoroughly discuss all the relevant issues, and work on some joint corrective exercises. This is **not** to deny that a **great deal** can be achieved by work on yourself, but it is fairly obvious that ultimately erectile confidence comes from gaining and maintaining erections during lovemaking with a partner. No matter how confident you eventually become about your ability to erect in private masturbation, there is often at the back of your mind uncertainty that it will also work with a partner.

Many impotent, partnerless males find themselves in a catch-22 situation: until they can find a caring partner with whom they can relate sexually quite comfortably, they cannot build up their sexual confidence. Because they lack sexual confidence, they find it very difficult to get into a non-threatening sexual situation with a partner. There are a number of solutions to this dilemma.

The first is to work with a professional surrogate partner — a trained woman who works with men to help them overcome their sexual difficulties. Most truly professional surrogates work in conjunction with, or only by referral from, a sex therapist, and it is from such a person that you would seek this kind of assistance. Note that professional surrogates are in no way, shape or form, prostitutes! Some few prostitutes are sympathetic to impotent men and will try to help them, but in general they will not, or lack the training which is necessary often for success.

Another solution is to form a relationship with a woman you like, and when you get to know her better, level with her about your difficulty. When you do, **describe the problem positively,** and

not apologetically! For example, you might say: 'I want you to know that I've had some minor problems getting and keeping an adequate erection, but I'm confident that as I get to know you better, and stop being worried about erections, these problems will go away. Anyway, I know it isn't necessary to have an erection to make love — we can be fully satisfied together, even without intercourse'. A new partner who does not respond sympathetically or helpfully to this type of up-front honest approach, is probably not going to have much to offer you in the long haul, and you might as well find out sooner rather than later! If you do get an unsympathetic response, **do not catastrophize** and convince yourself that **all** women will have the same response — this simply is not true! Just keep looking until you find the right partner!

My experience with many impotent men over the years has led me to have absolutely no doubt that the direct levelling approach just described is better than any other alternative with a new partner. It puts you into a no-lose situation! If she can't handle the situation sympathetically, she is not for you anyway, and you will find that out very quickly! More usually she will be accepting of the difficulty and try to help. Having levelled, you will find that you are much less anxious when you do get into the lovemaking situation with her. One further tip: say that you would like her to agree in advance, that at least for a little while, when you make love, no attempt at intercourse will be permitted, even if you happen to have a normal erection and feel very confident. Ask her not to give in, and to refuse intercourse, even if on the spur of the moment you change your mind and feel like giving it a try! By taking the pressure off your penis in this way, so that whether or not you erect is quite irrelevant, you will feel much less anxious. You can then really get to know your new partner sexually, at the same time thoroughly enjoying yourself and building up your sexual confidence. Some men I have worked with have found that they simply could not level this way with a new partner. Many of these clients have overcome their embarrassment and anxiety about levelling, by practising saying what needs to be said into a tape recorder. They then listen to what they have said, and then do it again, working to make it eventually sound just right for them, and continuing until they no longer feel uncomfortable saying it.

If, despite this practice, you still can't bring yourself to level, you might usefully resort to a harmless little white lie! Say something like this to your new partner, when it looks as though you are going to get into a sexual situation: 'By the way', (said as casually as possible), 'I recently injured my penis in a fall, and on medical advice I'm not allowed to have intercourse till it heals up. But that certainly won't stop me making love with you, and I'm sure we'll both have a wonderful time'. By thus stating up-front that intercourse is not going to occur, you remove from the lovemaking situation the dreadful anxiety about whether or not you will erect adequately. You can then enjoy yourself and gradually build up your confidence, simply allowing your penis to respond as it wishes.

You must remember that almost every person, man and woman alike, is a little anxious the first time they make love with a new partner — this is normal and virtually inevitable! To make sexual relating with a new partner as free from anxiety as possible, I have offered a few additional hints in appendix 16.

What if Nothing Can be Done to Restore Your Potency?

Sometimes, despite expert help, plus your own very best efforts, erectile impotence cannot be overcome, for a variety of possible reasons. Should this occur, it is not in any way the end of the world, **unless** you start catastrophizing and telling yourself over and over in your mind that you can never be happy, loved, or sexually fulfilled again!

You might consider a surgically implanted penile prosthesis, discussed earlier. This will certainly enable you to have normal intercourse. You must remember however, that intercourse is in no way essential for satisfying lovemaking, that women tend to be much less fussed about lack of erections than we men, and that you can almost always be manipulated to ejaculation and orgasm, without having an erection (see chapter 3). Many couples confronted with incurable impotence work out a perfectly satisfactory pattern of lovemaking without intercourse, culminating in mutual manipulation to orgasm. Surprisingly, some such couples report that their lovemaking is now much more exciting and satisfying than it was when intercourse was possible! This is because there is now on both sides much more emphasis on general body pleasuring and erotic stimulation. They have come to realize that when intercourse was possible, their main focus was on this, with neither partner putting much thought or effort into what they erroneously saw as mere preliminaries to the main event!

Some couples who cannot have normal intercourse, get extra pleasure from their lovemaking by learning how to 'stuff' the non-erect penis into the vagina. This technique, which sometimes takes a good deal of practice to master, involves the woman tucking the non-erect penis into her vagina, and is described in appendix 13. Some degree of thrusting may be possible, especially if the woman regularly exercises her pelvic muscles, and then uses them appropriately during penile movement.

While you are still actively trying to overcome impotence, perhaps hoping to find somewhere another therapist who can help you regain your potency, you simply **cannot** work at accepting your problem as a fact of life, and learning to make your sexual relationship with your partner as good as possible, in spite of this. In other words, while your goal is cure, it cannot be acceptance and adaptation! Many men with incurable impotence have reported that when they finally gave up trying to find a cure, and began for the first time to concentrate on acceptance, and making the best of the situation, they felt much happier and once again began to enjoy their sex life.

While reaching a climax when you make love is certainly not essential, it is often desired and enjoyable, and tends to relieve pent-up sexual tension. An erection is not necessary for achieving it, but should your partner have any difficulty in manipulating you to orgasm without an erection, the following suggestions may help.

1. Make sure your conditions for being sexually responsive are met (chapter 6).
2. Get your partner to anchor your penis at its base, by holding

it with her left hand (or right, if she is left-handed). This prevents it wobbling too much. With the same hand, get her also to hold **all** the loose skin of the penis **firmly** down at its base. If she does not, then as her right hand tries to manipulate your penis, she will merely move loose skin up and down over the shaft of the penis, which does not provide much stimulation. When the loose skin is firmly anchored at the base of the penis, much more friction and therefore stimulation is possible. Her left hand can also gently compress the base of the penis, acting like a tourniquet.

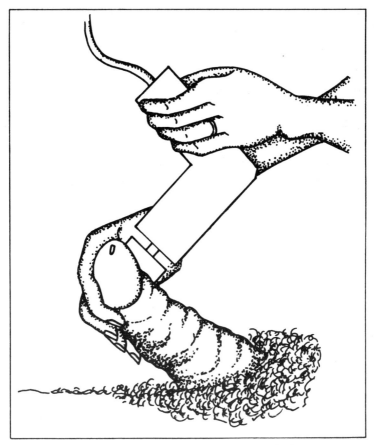

Fig. 7 Correct use of a mains-operated electrical vibrator to assist ejaculation without an erection

3. Make sure your penis and her right hand are adequately lubricated (try warmed-up baby oil).

4. Make sure she stimulates the penis **vigorously** with her right hand — many women are far too gentle, erroneously fearing that they will hurt their partner. Consider using the position suggested in appendix 13, for the first step of the joint erectile exercises, as it is often the most comfortable for your partner, and gives her the best possible access to your whole genital area.

5. Give her feedback, and instructions about exactly what kind of stimulation you need, and precisely where you want it.

6. Do **not** make the mistake of **working at climaxing,** of actively **trying** to make yourself ejaculate!

7. Experiment to see whether contracting and relaxing your pelvic muscles and/or your buttock muscles gives you more arousal. Some men get most aroused from penile stimulation when they deliberately hold their pelvic and/or buttock muscles firmly tensed. If you do deliberately tense these muscles, make **absolutely sure** you are not then making the mistake of trying to reach a climax!

8. Increase your arousal by any means that is effective for you. For example, fondle her breasts or genitals, tune into an arousing fantasy, and so on.

9. If despite the above suggestions, you feel you still need extra stimulation to reach orgasm, you could use an electric vibrator. The best type is mains-operated and has an attachment on which the penis is placed, at the junction of the head (glans) and shaft, as is shown in figure 7.

   The penis needs to be held gently against the vibrator attachment by several fingers. Some experimentation may be needed to work out what is for you the best way of using the vibrator. Battery-operated penis-shaped vibrators are usually not particularly effective for men who find it difficult to ejaculate.

Should you not have a partner, and experience difficulty in masturbating to orgasm, you can of course adapt these suggestions to provide yourself with effective stimulation.

Appendix 1

AN APPROACH TO HELP DEVELOP THE KEY SEXUAL ATTITUDE

The crucial attitude, which you **must** work at developing, is simply this: **lovemaking means just that, and an erect penis and intercourse are not in any way necessary for it!**

The facts that most men find this notion a little unusual at first glance, and that more often than not for most people lovemaking does involve an erect penis and intercourse, **do not in any way invalidate this notion!**

Why is this Attitude so Important?

Apart from being absolutely true, it is the basis of ongoing, lifelong sexual happiness, for both males and females. When you really believe and accept it, for the first time sexual expression becomes relieved of performance concerns which cause so much misery for so many people! As you are painfully aware, anxiety about getting and keeping an adequate erection is grossly destructive to a man's actual erectile ability!

A General Principle about Attitude Change

Well established, entrenched beliefs are notoriously difficult to alter! Reading about more appropriate attitudes, and logical argument, are not particularly effective in changing one's established beliefs. In general, the most effective and quickest way to change an attitude, is to **change behaviour** — in other words, to actually **do** certain things relevant to the attitudes it is desired to change and acquire.

Some 'Doing' Things to Help Develop the Key Sexual Attitude

1. Make love as often as you feel like, but **under no circumstances** attempt vaginal penetration, even if you have a perfectly normal erection!

2. As often as you get a chance, engage in some form of gentle, direct sexual touching with your partner, in situations where there is no chance of the contact progressing to formal lovemaking. For example, when kissing her goodbye as you leave for work, lovingly fondle her breasts and genitals through her clothes, and ask her to do the same for you. Just concentrate on enjoying what you are doing and experiencing, for the pleasure of the moment.

3. **Every time** you catch yourself thinking that without an adequate erection you are no good, or inadequate as a man, or unable to fully satisfy your partner, or similar irrational and destructive thoughts, put a cross on a small note pad which you carry around at all times for this specific purpose. Do this **immediately** you become aware that you are having the unwanted thought. This is a very effective procedure called 'self-monitoring', and if you do it **exactly** as described, the frequency with which you experience these thoughts will steadily decrease. Simple, isn't it!

4. While giving your partner a non-sexual cuddle in private, explain to her **in full detail** exactly how you feel emotionally when during lovemaking with her you can't get or hold an erection. Explain just how your anxiety, shame and so on, affects you, what sort of thoughts you have, what you fear she may be thinking, what you fear she may do, what you fear the future may hold. As you elaborate on these emotions and irrational thoughts, keep telling her (and yourself!) just how ridiculous it

is for you to think and feel this way, and how grossly you tend to exaggerate the importance of an adequate erection. Do this as often as possible, whenever you get the chance!

By thus repeatedly expressing your fears, and ridiculing them, you will find that they will decrease. Sharing them with your partner will also help her to understand and assist you. Note that you are only ridiculing your ideas and beliefs, **not** yourself — **you are not under any circumstances putting yourself down!**

5. With your partner's help, work out and write down a comprehensive and very detailed list of all the specific advantages (for you, her, and you both) of lovemaking not having to involve intercourse, or any other specific goal. These will mainly revolve around:

   a. Eradicating all anxiety or concern about sexual performance, allowing you both to simply enjoy yourself and each other.
   b. Encouraging you to try new forms of stimulation and develop an entirely new approach to sensuality.

   Be **very specific** as you list these advantages — for example:

   a. We can make love when we feel interested, without having to worry about whether or not I will get an erection.
   b. We can make love without me having to worry about whether or not I will be able to bring you to orgasm.
   c. We can still make love when I feel tired, without me having to worry that I might perhaps go to sleep during lovemaking.

   Having worked out this list, put it away, and a day or so later begin **thoroughly** discussing each item with your partner, over a number of short sessions.

6. Teach as many other people as possible (friends, adult children, workmates) that lovemaking means just that, and there is absolutely **no** element of performance — **it is always a success!** When doing this, of course, you certainly don't have to reveal that you have an erection problem! It could be worthwhile, however, saying that with your partner, no one fusses if you start lovemaking and wind up going to sleep before you have got a proper erection, or something similar.

The general principle is that teaching someone else a new attitude, is an excellent and powerful way of developing it yourself!

7. This will sound totally ridiculous, but it is **very** useful and effective — give it a try!

   In private, close your eyes, and imagine yourself in a sexual situation with your partner, unable to erect. Then imagine yourself being **very anxious.** Then, **out loud,** talk to your (imaginary) anxiety as if it were a naughty child! Scold it, ridicule it, forbid it, and so on. Refer to it by name — for example:

   'Anxiety, you are a stupid, miserable, inconsiderate spoil-sport! How dare you come into my mind — take yourself off and get out of my hair. You're crazy if you think I'm going to let you interfere with me making love, with or without an erection!' Put some **real feeling** into what you are saying, and keep the whole process up for as long as possible, but at least 2 minutes. Do this repeatedly, on the basis that 'a little often is best'. The more stupid you feel doing this, the more effective the technique!

8. If you thought manoeuvre 7 was ridiculous, you will think this one is absolutely crazy, but do it anyway! When you have time to practise, go and sit on the lid of your toilet, in private. Then 'worry out loud' in an exaggerated manner, about not being able to get or keep an adequate erection during lovemaking. Try to **make yourself genuinely upset** about your erectile problem, for example, by saying **with artificially contrived feeling** if need be, things like:

   'I'll **never** be able to have sex again: it's the **end** of the world for me: no woman will **ever** want to have **anything** to do with me **ever** again: it is the **most terrible** thing **ever** to happen to me', and so on. Make these statements as **exaggerated and extreme** as possible. **Force** yourself to keep going until you just can't generate **any** more emotions, no matter how hard you try — **this is very important!** Do **not** stop this exercise until you are quite literally unable to continue! It is even more effective, should you have the facilities, to tape record your 'out-loud exaggerated worrying' and, as soon as you have finished, **immediately** force yourself to listen to the tape! If you can overcome your feelings of seeming like an idiot, and listen to this tape with your partner, it will be even more useful!

Should you feel absolutely stupid about this whole procedure, first say to yourself several times, out loud **with feeling:** 'Williams is insane but I'll humour him by doing this crazy exercise'. Remember, the more ridiculous you actually feel, the **more effective** the procedure.

Repeat this exercise as often as possible, until you are **certain** that your attitudes have changed!

9. Use the Premack principle, as described in appendix 2.

10. Use autosuggestion, as described in appendix 9.

You may wonder why I have offered so many different manoeuvres to help you develop the key sexual attitude. My reasons are simple — you **must** develop this attitude; achieving it is not exactly a push-over; and not every self-help technique works properly for each and every person.

If you accept my view that you **must** develop this attitude, **force** yourself to do as many of these 'doing' exercises as possible, even if you feel uncomfortable or totally stupid! If **after a fair trial,** one of these approaches somehow just doesn't seem to be helpful for you, stop doing it!

You will know when you can stop working on acquiring this key attitude — it will seem perfectly natural to you, and you will no longer be concerned or anxious about whether or not you erect!

Appendix 2

THE USE OF THE PREMACK PRINCIPLE

This is used here as a simple, ingenious and effective means of changing unwanted attitudes. In essence, you **force** yourself repeatedly to think whatever it is you want to believe, **with feeling,** when you are reminded to do so by some frequently occurring activity in your daily life. One of the beauties of this technique is that it is effective **even if** you currently believe the exact opposite of the attitude you are working at acquiring!

Memorize this statement, word for word:

Good, satisfying lovemaking does not necessarily have to involve intercourse, and certainly does not require an erection — with or without an erection, lovemaking is always a success!

Next, work out some frequently recurring event in your daily routine, for example, making a telephone call. **Force** yourself to say or think the above statement, **with the maximum possible feeling,** 6 times **before** you allow yourself to make each and every phone call. If you can't think of anything that happens frequently, link the statement to **water** — i.e. **before** you allow yourself to **touch** water, **drink** water (which means any liquid at all) or **pass** water (urinate), **first** you say or think the statement 6 times, **with maximum feeling!**

You will find that if you do this simple manoeuvre regularly for a few weeks, it will greatly assist you in acquiring the desired attitude to your sexual expression. Keep using this procedure until you are **quite convinced** that the desired attitude is **truly** now your own.

Even though this sounds extremely simple, and is totally contrived, you will find it **very helpful** indeed!

While initially you will probably use this to help you acquire the key sexual attitude described, you can subsequently use it to help overcome the destructive effects of other persistent unwanted attitudes, based on other sexual myths.

Appendix 3

THOUGHT STOPPING

This is a simple and effective psychological procedure for getting unwanted thoughts out of one's mind, and there are a number of different ways of doing it. The variation to be described is particularly effective in getting rid of unwanted thoughts when you are in a sexual situation.

The Procedure

Say out loud, or if that is not possible, think to yourself:

'Stop: I'm not going to let myself think like that: it's irrational'.

Then, immediately imagine yourself in a standard, peaceful, relaxing scene, for 3 seconds. While doing this, close your eyes if that is possible. If you can't, think of your peaceful scene with your eyes open, for 3 seconds.

Some Important Points

1. Always use **exactly** the same words — do not change them in any way!
2. Wear a thick elastic band on your wrist, and as you think 'stop', give yourself a **really painful** flick on the wrist. If that is not possible, because it would be embarrassing, bite your tongue or cheek! This painful stimulus as you think 'stop', will enable you

to learn this technique **much** more rapidly. Of course, when you are absolutely expert at thought stopping, it will no longer be necessary to give yourself a painful stimulus.

3. **Always** say or think this sequence with **plenty of feeling or emphasis!** Unless this is done, each and every time you use thought stopping, it will not work properly. **Never** allow the thought stopping sequence to become an unemotional, neutral series of words!

4. Say or think this sequence at normal talking speed — do **not** go through it too rapidly!

5. Always use **exactly** the same peaceful scene! Repeatedly practise visualizing it, until it is always the same.

6. It will require perhaps several thousand practice runs, until this technique is fully effective in getting rid of unwanted thoughts. Whatever you do, **don't make the mistake** of giving up because it hasn't worked properly after only a few hundred trials!

How to Practise Thought Stopping

1. Wear a thick elastic band on the wrist on which you wear your watch. Whenever you look at the time, you will see the elastic band, and this will remind you to practise your thought stopping technique.

2. For a few days, only use thought stopping against trivial passing thoughts which are of no importance to you, until the technique becomes automatic. When you can do it without having to think about it, do two things:
   a. Keep practising on any trivial thoughts which come into your mind, whenever you think of it. The elastic band will help to remind you to do this.
   b. Start using it against thoughts which you genuinely wish to be rid of for some reason, such as worrying or upsetting thoughts. When you start doing this, you will naturally find that as soon as you have finished the thought stopping sequence, the unwanted thoughts will come back. You then immediately repeat the whole sequence, performing this over and over again, if necessary, to keep the unwanted thoughts

out of your mind. Even though doing this repeatedly is boring, you will have no alternative for a while. However, each time you do it over and over again, the effectiveness of the procedure will slowly and progressively increase.

Caution
Always put some feeling or emphasis into your thought stopping sequence, no matter how many thousands of times you might have done it! **Never,** under any circumstances, allow the sequence to become mechanical or unemotional!

How to Use Thought Stopping

1. Outside the sexual situation
You **must** declare **war** on thoughts about your sexual performance, regardless of the circumstances under which they occur! In **any** situation, **the instant** you realize that you are thinking about your sexual performance, push these grossly destructive thoughts out of your mind, using thought stopping, repeating it over and over again if need be.

2. In a Sexual Situation

Here it is **absolutely essential** to rid your mind of any unhelpful thoughts! These might be thoughts about your sexual performance (for example: 'I hope I will get hard enough'), or thoughts about unrelated matters, such as an unresolved problem from work.

There is a simple variation on your standard thought stopping technique, which is often **even more useful** when you are in physical contact with your partner. It goes like this: **'Stop: I'm not going to let myself think like that: it's irrational: all I have to do is concentrate on what I'm feeling now'.** Then, concentrate all your attention on the physical sensations you experience, as you are touched, or as you touch your partner.

You can practise this variation of the standard thought stopping procedure, on either trivial or genuinely unwanted thoughts, **after** you have mastered the basic technique. When you do practise, touch yourself and concentrate on the sensations you experience. When you feel proficient, practise when you are touching, or being touched by, your partner in a non-sexual setting, for example if you are holding hands while you watch TV.

Remember

1. You **must** declare war on unhelpful thoughts, **especially** thoughts about your sexual performance, past, present or future!
2. Until you are truly expert at this procedure, you may have to do thought stopping over and over again, to keep unwanted thoughts out of your mind. However, this is infinitely better than allowing yourself repeatedly to think destructive thoughts!
3. You **must** always use some feeling or emphasis, each and every time you do thought stopping!
4. If you just keep practising over and over again, you **must eventually** develop a powerful and effective skill for getting rid of any kind of unwanted thoughts, not just ones related to sex!

Note

If you have difficulty **visualizing** a peaceful scene in your mind, you might try one of the following alternatives:
1. Visualize instead, a blank white wall or a STOP sign.
2. Play in your head a brief segment of your favourite music, making it always the same.

Appendix 4

SENSUALITY TRAINING EXERCISES

Step 1 Learning to Focus on Skin Sensations

Close your eyes, and touch yourself on some exposed part of your body. See if you can focus mentally on the temperature — is it warm or cold? Then focus on the pressure feeling — is it light or firm? Then focus on the texture — is it smooth or rough? Finally, focus on the presence or absence of moisture — is it absolutely dry or is there some moisture present?

Practise this for only 10 to 20 seconds at a time, whenever you think of it, until it is very easy for you to quickly focus mentally on these four basic sensations, one after the other, whenever you touch yourself on any part of your body.

When you have become proficient at doing this, take it a step further, and learn to 'lose yourself' in the sensations you are feeling as you touch yourself with your eyes closed. This means learning to concentrate on these feelings to such an extent that you are **totally unaware of anything else** — in other words, you have no thoughts about any other thing, no awareness of anything around you. You will find that mastering this skill takes quite a lot of practice, so don't be discouraged when it turns out to be harder than you think! Practise for several minutes at a time, as often as possible.

When you have **thoroughly** mastered these basic skills, then, and only then, progress to step 2.

Step 2 Focusing on and Losing Yourself in Other Sensations

Gather together some articles with a different feel, such as fur, velvet, feathers, plastic, butter, an orange and so on. With your eyes closed, practise lightly touching these while you focus mentally on the physical sensations produced. Once again, aim to 'lose yourself' in the feelings, so that you have all your mental processes focused on the sensations you are experiencing, to the complete exclusion of everything else. See if you can hold this exclusive focus for a few minutes at a time. Repeat this exercise using different materials, doing it as often as possible.

Step 3 Verbalizing Physical Sensations

Repeat step 2, using a variety of different objects, but now say out loud to yourself exactly what you are feeling! You will discover that it is not easy to put words to physical sensations, and that considerable frequent practice is required. Nonetheless, the effort is more than worth while, as the skills involved are extremely important for maximizing your potential for arousal during sexual contact.

Step 4 Losing Yourself in Visual, Olfactory (Smell) Gustatory (Taste) and Auditory (Hearing) Sensations

Select some printed scene or picture, or some pleasant looking object. Then, close your eyes, and visualize it in your mind's eye. Learn to 'lose yourself' in this mental picture — focus all your thought processes on it, so that you are aware of nothing else. See if you can learn to hold this internal visual concentration for a few minutes at a time.

When you can easily do this, master the same skill using the other kinds of sensations. **With your eyes closed,** focus on a pleasant smell, and try to hold on to this alone, so that you are aware of nothing else. Do the same with an agreeable taste in your mouth, and finally with some appealing music or other sound.

A common response to my suggesting these exercises is that they are stupid (and Williams is mad!). While, as always, you are entitled to your own view, my experience, both personally, and in my efforts to help sexually dysfunctional people, has convinced me of 2 things:

1. Most people do not know how to focus on and lose themselves in pleasant sensations.
2. The ability to focus on and lose oneself in pleasant sensations is one of the most important skills needed in overcoming sexual problems and in maximizing one's sexual potential!

I don't ask you to believe me, but I do ask that you give me the benefit of the doubt and diligently practise what I have asked! If you do this conscientiously and thoroughly you will find that a whole new dimension of physical awareness is opened up to you, and that this will enhance both your sexual enjoyment and your erectile potency.

Do yourself a favour and give all these exercises a damn good try!

Appendix 5

SELF RELAXATION

*Why You Should Master Skills in Relaxation if
You are Impotent*

1. You can't afford to be anxious or tense in a sexual situation, if you are to have a chance of erecting adequately.
2. You can't be simultaneously anxious and relaxed! They are incompatible states and cannot co-occur, just as you can't have ice floating around in boiling water! You can therefore use relaxation to get rid of anxiety and tension.
3. If you feel that life generally is stressful, you can use regular formal relaxation as a way of reducing the harmful effects of this stress. The effects of stress, you will recall, were described in chapter 8.

How to Relax Yourself

I am going to describe two unrelated methods, as different individuals often find one or the other more effective, or more suitable for their own particular circumstances.

Method 1   Progressive Muscular Relaxation

Practise this lying down in a comfortable position, eyes closed, clothing completely loose (for example, shoes off, tie off, belt undone). Let your breathing come and go as it chooses — **do not deliberately breathe deeply or in any particular way!**

Focus mentally on your feet — visualize them in your mind's eye, or simply think of them. Then, deliberately tense the muscles of your feet, making them as tight as possible without causing any discomfort. **Try to do this without actually moving your feet.** When these muscles are as tight as you can comfortably make them, just let go and **allow** them to completely relax. As you let them relax, repeatedly **think** to yourself, silently in your mind, each time you breathe out, 'relax'.

When the feet muscles feel completely relaxed, stop thinking 'relax' as you breathe out, and focus mentally on your calf muscles. Tense them as much as you can comfortably, without actually moving your legs. When they are as tense as you can comfortably make them, just let go of the tension, again thinking to yourself, silently in your mind, each time you breathe out, 'relax'.

When the calf muscles feel fully relaxed, repeat the process with your thigh muscles, then your stomach muscles, then your neck muscles, then your jaw muscles, then your forehead muscles, then your arm muscles, then your forearm and hand muscles. When your hand muscles have been allowed to relax, pretend that you are in a standard imaginary peaceful scene, for example, lying on a beach, and keep thinking 'relax' as you breathe out. Continue imagining yourself in this scene, thinking 'relax' as you breathe out, for about a minute.

You should find that initially this exercise takes about 10 to 15 minutes. Once you've got the hang of doing it, so you don't have to think much about what you do next, or how you do it, you will find that at the end of the exercise, you will feel relaxed, increasingly so with repeated practice.

Always imagine exactly the same peaceful scene at the end — this is **very** important! With repeated practice of the exercise, that standard scene will become a trigger signal to relax. Then, when you imagine it, and repeatedly think 'relax' as you breathe out, without any preliminary muscle tensing and relaxing, you will very quickly become relaxed.

With regular practice, you can eventually run through the whole exercise in about 7 minutes. If possible, practise twice daily until you have thoroughly mastered it, and additionally can quickly relax yourself, simply by thinking 'relax' as you breathe out, and imagining your peaceful scene. You can then scale down the practice, and maintain your relaxation skills by doing the actual exercise once or twice per week, most conveniently in bed, just before you go to sleep at night.

To get rid of anxiety or tension during lovemaking, or in any other situation, simply close your eyes, imagine yourself in your standard peaceful scene, and think 'relax' each time you breathe out. If you can't close your eyes, think of yourself in your standard peaceful scene with your eyes open, and keep thinking 'relax' each time you breathe out.

Method 2   A Breathing Technique

Practise seated comfortably in a chair with your head hanging forward, or lying down. Close your eyes and focus mentally on your lower chest and upper stomach.

Take a **very** shallow breath in, **thinking** silently in your mind, 'one'. Then, take an equally shallow breath out, also thinking 'one'. Make your next breath in also shallow, but **just a little deeper,** thinking 'one and two'. Then, breathe out, also thinking 'one and two'. The next breath in will be **just a little deeper,** and you will think 'one and two and three'; the same when you breathe out. The next breath in and out will be a little deeper, as you think one to four, the next even deeper as you think one to five, and so on, until you finally reach **the very deepest breath** you can take. When this has occurred, on your **next** breath in, go right back to the beginning of this sequence. In other words, take a **very** shallow breath in and out, thinking 'one', and repeat the sequence, progressively increasing the depth of breathing up to your maximum. Continue thus for about 3 to 5 minutes, but don't formally time yourself by using a watch — just guess when the practice time is up.

You will find that it takes a little while to get the hang of breathing this way, but it is not really difficult. When you can breathe this way without having to think too much about it, you will find yourself beginning to relax.

You will discover that with repeated practice, you can breathe this way, and quickly relax yourself, **without having to think the numbers.** You should certainly practise until you can in fact easily do this, even with your eyes open.

Practise for up to 5 minutes at a time, as often as you can, until you can quickly relax yourself using this procedure — within 1 to 2 minutes. When you can do this, maintain your skill by practising for a few minutes, just before you go to sleep at night, several times each week.

If you feel anxious or tense during lovemaking, or in any other situation, use this breathing technique to quickly relax away the unwanted feelings, repeating it should they recur. With diligent practice, this should eventually be quite easy to achieve.

Note

You can of course, use relaxation skills to combat 'uptight' feelings other than anxiety, such as anger.

Appendix 6

PELVIC MUSCLE EXERCISE

This exercise will develop and strengthen those muscles in and around your pelvis which are extremely important for your optimal sexual functioning. With regular practice, it may improve your erectile performance, and should make your experience of orgasm more pleasurable. It may even lead to you developing the ability to have multiple orgasms!

Step 1

When you urinate, practise repeatedly stopping and starting the stream of urine. When you can easily do this, learn to do it **without in any way using your stomach muscles!** Put one hand firmly over your lower abdomen to make sure these muscles are not moving to assist in stopping the flow of urine.

Step 2

When the first step has been mastered, practise exactly the same movement, when you are not urinating. Practise 10 times in a row, 3 times daily. Gradually, over a few weeks, steadily increase, until you can do it approximately 100 times in a row, 3 times daily. It is a good idea to discipline yourself to do this exercise each time you have a meal. This will remind you to do it, and as it is an exercise you will hopefully do for **the rest of your life,** it will become an automatic routine at meal times.

Remember

1. Make sure you do **not** use your stomach muscles!
2. Increase the number of repetitions **gradually** from 10 to 100, over a few weeks.
3. Practise 3 times daily, **forever!**
4. It may take a month or two before you start to notice benefits from the increased muscle strength.

Appendix 7

FANTASY TRAINING

A fantasy is just a series of thoughts about some imaginary subject — in other words, a daydream. All normal people engage in fantasy thinking from time to time, and this is both healthy and desirable. Some daydreams or fantasies are about sexual subjects, and likewise all normal people have them from time to time. For example, if while lazing in the sun at the beach you have sexual thoughts about some attractive woman you are watching, this is a sexual fantasy, and is perfectly normal.

You may be surprised to know that many **women** frequently engage in some form of sexual fantasy **during lovemaking.** There is, of course, **absolutely nothing wrong** with this, and it is an activity frankly to be **encouraged!** We men tend to use fantasy **during lovemaking** far less, until perhaps problems arise.

You will find that if you learn how to use sexual fantasies to your advantage during lovemaking, it will be easier to erect and maintain your erection. You will also be less likely to be troubled by unhelpful thoughts, for example, about whether or not you will get an adequate erection. However, before you can benefit fully from the use of fantasy during lovemaking, you need to know a few facts, and to do some practice!

Relevant Facts

1. The kinds of sexual fantasy that are arousing to different individuals (both men and women) are extremely variable. Some are very turned on by imagining sexual activities which other equally normal people find offputting, or even frankly revolting. Remember, one man's meat is another man's poison! **The crucial thing to understand is that whatever sexual imaginings turn you on, that is normal and fine!** Only actual 'doing' behaviour can be abnormal, and **there is a world of difference between imagining something and actually doing it!**

2. There is absolutely no reason to feel guilty if you are imagining some form of sexual activity with another person, during lovemaking with your partner. **It does not in any way mean that you don't love her, or that you really would prefer someone else!** It is **not** 'mental adultery' — it is simply a useful and enjoyable form of sexual behaviour!

3. There is no particular reason why you should tell your partner, during or after lovemaking, that you are or were using a sexual fantasy, or what it was. What goes on in the privacy of your mind is your business and you are **not** in any way obligated to reveal it to anyone! Of course, there is equally no reason why you should not reveal your fantasies to your partner, if you choose. Many sophisticated lovers find that sharing their fantasies, during or after lovemaking, heightens their arousal and enjoyment, and brings them even closer emotionally, because of this very intimate form of sharing.

4. You simply can't expect to get the full benefit from the use of fantasy during lovemaking, until you have practised and developed the skill! After all, you have to learn to be quite comfortable within yourself doing this, and you have to master the skill of engaging in a pleasurable fantasy at the same time as you actually make love with your partner, and also focus on your own physical sensations, especially those from your genitals. It is something like learning to play 3 musical instruments, all at the same time!

How to Learn to Use Fantasy to Your Advantage During Lovemaking

1. In private, think of the most exciting imaginary sexual situations you can possibly dream up. Let your imagination have a field day, bearing in mind that **in fantasy absolutely anything goes!** Make a note of the kinds of sexual activities and situations you find most arousing. If you want some ideas, read one of the books on sexual fantasy listed in appendix 18.

2. Next, in private, while seated or lying, select one of your exciting imaginary sexual situations, and with your eyes closed, develop an **ongoing** fantasy in your mind. This will be a story **involving you,** with a beginning, a middle and an end. Make sure it lasts at the very least for a few minutes. **As you fantasize, try to pretend that it is actually happening to you now!** If you have difficulty fantasizing in this way, it may help to start by looking at some erotic pictures, or by reading some appropriately arousing material. Once you are into the swing of it, you can then close your eyes to develop your own mental pictures. With practice, you will find you no longer need any aid to begin vivid fantasizing.

   Repeat this exercise as often as possible, using in sequence several of the different fantasy situations and activities that most appeal to you. Remember, do a little often, rather than spend a long time at this task infrequently! Should you have difficulty **visualizing** an appealing fantasy in your mind, you might try imagining the **physical sensations** that accompany the thoughts that make up the fantasy.

3. When it is easy to run through a small repertoire of arousing fantasies in your mind, in private, begin using them during lovemaking. Remember, it takes **some considerable practice** to be able to concentrate on a fantasy while you are making love, and also focus on your genital feelings! It often helps to pretend that the sensations you are actually experiencing are really being produced by whatever is happening in the fantasy, this being especially important if you find it hard to actually visualize it in your mind.

You will probably find it easiest and most effective to use those fantasies which you have been rehearsing in private. Should you feel a little uncomfortable, perhaps even guilty, about using fantasies during lovemaking with your partner, **simply press on!** You will find that the inappropriate and completely irrational anxiety or guilt feelings will soon disappear with continued practice.

You will find that the deliberate use of rehearsed sexual fantasy is combined with some of the exercises specifically directed at overcoming your problem.

Appendix 8

DESENSITIZATION

This is a simple and effective technique for overcoming your anxiety, guilt and so on, about the possibility that you will not achieve or maintain an adequate erection in the sexual situation. You should practise it if, despite mastering and using thought stopping and relaxation, and avoiding all attempts at intercourse during lovemaking, you are still aware of being **in any way** nervous, anxious or uneasy when you make love with your partner, or in anticipation of doing so.

The principle of desensitization is very simple: If, **while deeply relaxed,** you repeatedly **imagine** some situation which in real life makes you inappropriately anxious (or guilty, ashamed and so on!), you will gradually and progressively cease being inappropriately anxious (or guilty etc.) in the real life situation.

How to Perform Desensitization

First, work out and write down a series of **brief** scenes, covering typical examples of past actual sexual situations where you have had erection problems. Write these in the present tense, as though they were actually happening now.

For example:

1. 'I am making love with Mary: she is very aroused and wanting penetration, but I haven't got an adequate erection.'

2. 'I am making love with Mary: I have just penetrated her and my erection is going down — she is obviously very disappointed'.

Keep each scene as short as in my examples, and do **not** include in the scene how **you** felt. For example, do **not** say '. . . and I feel very nervous, guilty and humiliated'.

Make sure you include in your list of scenes examples of **all** the various situations in which you have **ever** had erection problems. These might include during masturbation, with various previous partners, in different kinds of sexual activities with a particular partner, and so on. The general rule is to **be comprehensive** — it is better to have too many scenes rather than too few!

Next, work out and write down a similar series of scenes, this time covering **possible future situations,** which you have not actually experienced, but which you could **perhaps** encounter some time in the future, and which would make you anxious, guilty and so on, were they to happen now.

This is **especially important** if currently you do not have a regular partner.

For example:

1. 'I am making love with Mary: she is orally stimulating my penis: it is remaining completely limp: she is obviously frustrated'.
2. 'I am making love with a new partner for the first time. She is very aroused and wanting penetration, but in spite of her fondling me, I haven't got even the beginning of an erection: she is puzzled and upset'.

Next, having worked out your list of scenes (usually 10 to 30 as a rough guide), write them down on small cards (say about the size of an appointment card), **one scene per card.** You are now ready to begin practising desensitization, and here is how you proceed:

1. Lie down in private in a quiet place, where you will not be disturbed. Have your pile of cards nearby so they can be easily turned up, one at a time, and read. The pile of cards can be in **any order.** They do **not,** for example, have to be in sequence from the first time the problem occured, through to the present and then the future.

2. Relax yourself with your eyes closed, using one of the techniques suggested earlier. When you feel reasonably relaxed, gently, without losing your relaxation, turn up the first card and read it. Then, put it down separate from the main pile, close your eyes again, and try to imagine whatever situation was described on that card. **Do your best to pretend that whatever was described is actually happening now!** Do **not** just vaguely remember it, or see it in your mind as though you were watching it happen on a movie screen. **As soon as you are aware that in any way you are beginning to lose your relaxation, stop imagining, and re-relax yourself.** Do **not** wait until imagining the situation makes you actually anxious, uneasy, tense or uncomfortable! Stop imagining **at the very first sign** that you are **starting** to lose your relaxation!   ·

3. When you again feel reasonably relaxed, re-imagine the **same** scene, **as though it were actually happening.** Stop imagining it, and again relax yourself at the **first sign** of loss of relaxation. Repeat this process with the **same scene,** until imagining it vividly, as though it were actually happening, simply does not concern you **in any way at all!** When you can do this with the scene on the first card, move to the second card, doing the same thing. Should any scene **not** cause you to lose your feeling of relaxation, the very first time you imagine it vividly, proceed directly to the next card.

4. If possible, perform this procedure for about 20 minutes each practice session, but certainly for no longer. If however you can only manage perhaps 10-15 minutes, this is still worthwhile. A lesser period than 10 minutes is not practicable.

    It is quite possible that in a single practice session, you may not become totally comfortable repeatedly imagining one particular scene. It may still cause you to lose your relaxation by the end of the session. Should this occur, simply resume the next practice period using the same scene.

5. Repeat this exercise, if possible on a daily or even twice daily basis, until you have worked through the entire pack of cards, so that when you imagine them, **none** of the scenes in any

way causes you to begin to lose your relaxation. When you have finished the first run through all the cards, start again from the beginning, just to be **absolutely** sure that none of the scenes worries you in **any** way!

When you have completely and correctly finished this exercise, you will find that your feelings of anxiety, guilt and so on, about your erectile problem, have disappeared, or are **very much** less!

Note

You can also use desensitization to help overcome irrational feelings of anxiety, anger, guilt, shame, disgust or jealousy, **of any origin,** which may be contributing to your erectile problem.

Appendix 9

AUTOSUGGESTION

We are all suggestible — that is, affected by what other people say to us, and by the things we say to ourselves. In a relaxed state, where our mind can more easily focus on what is being said or thought, we are much more suggestible than usual, and therefore more powerfully affected by what is said or by our own thoughts.

It is easy enough to exploit your own suggestibility to your advantage, by repeatedly giving yourself appropriate suggestions, in a situation where these will have their maximum impact. The procedure is very simple, and I recommend its use to help you change and overcome the effects of unhelpful attitudes, based on sexual myths, interfering with your erectile ability.

How Do You Do It?

1. Sit comfortably in a chair, eyes closed, head slightly forward.
2. Relax yourself using one or other of the methods described in appendix 5.
3. Think to yourself, **slowly and with feeling,** the appropriate suggestion, which you must first have memorized, word for word.

    For example, to help develop the key sexual attitude (appendix 1), you might use the following:

    'Lovemaking is **just a way of showing love:** an erection **is totally unnecessary:** Lovemaking is **always a success!'**

4. Repeat the suggestion **6 times, with feeling,** then remain relaxed for about half a minute before opening your eyes. Stay seated for a further minute before you get up.

Do this simple little exercise as often as you can — with practice it will only take 3 to 4 minutes. Aim to do it **at least** 3 times daily, and **continue until you are completely confident that the desired attitude is yours!**

You can use this technique to help overcome the effects of any destructive sexual myth, but use it to tackle **only one** particular myth at a time! Wait until you feel your new attitude has been **set in concrete** before using autosuggestion against another sexual myth.

Hints on Wording Suggestions

1. Keep them **short** and **simple** — as though talking to a child!
2. Try to word the suggestion **positively,** and avoid negative words such as 'no', 'not' and so on.

   For example, do **not** say something like this: 'I do not have to have an erection to make love: even without it, lovemaking can still be successful'. Note that the overall tone of this suggestion is **negative.** You would have turned it into a **positive suggestion,** if you changed it to this: 'An erection is totally unnecessary during lovemaking and lovemaking is always a success'.

   With a little practice, **any** suggestion can be worded **positively!**
3. Always **write down** the suggestion you propose to use, and then check to make sure the above two rules have been obeyed. When you have got it right (short, simple and positive), **memorize it,** word for word, **before** using it in this exercise.
4. Use only **one suggestion** each time. Don't get ambitious and attempt to give yourself several suggestions when you use this technique.

Note

You can also use autosuggestion to combat irrational attitudes causing anger, guilt and so on.

Appendix 10

INDIVIDUAL ERECTILE EXERCISES

Some General Rules for Doing these Important Exercises

1. **You need good conditions!** You must have guaranteed privacy and freedom from interruption, and your 'conditions for being responsive' (chapter 6) must be met. If you have difficulty obtaining good circumstances under which to practise, your first task will be to rearrange your daily/weekly schedule so that you can! When there is a real will to succeed, you will find a way around problems, whatever the difficulties!
2. You **must** get into a sensual frame of mind **first!** There is no point trying these exercises immediately you finish some unrelated chore. You might, for example, listen to your favourite music for a while, read or look at erotic material for a time, or perhaps enjoy a relaxed bath.
3. During the exercises, you **must concentrate on the physical sensations you are experiencing!** If necessary, use thought stopping to get rid of thoughts about **anything** else. In those exercises where you are required also to fantasize, you must still try to concentrate on your genital feelings. This takes a bit of practice, but it can be done! It may help to pretend that the feelings you are actually experiencing in your genitals, are being produced by whatever is happening in the fantasy.
4. Strictly avoid **trying** to make anything happen! Remember, if

you try to make yourself erect, you will make your problem worse, not better!

5. Make haste slowly! Do not move from one step to the next until you are **absolutely** sure you have mastered the goals of the present step. **The commonest error that men make, is trying to go too fast!**

6. In all the steps, do **not** begin touching yourself on your genitals as soon as you start the exercise! First, 'warm up', by pleasurably stroking **other parts of your body,** focusing on what you then feel. Make sure you are **completely relaxed** before you begin the genital touching part of the exercises. If necessary, use one of the formal quick relaxation methods, described in appendix 5.

7. You must not ejaculate/have an orgasm during or after these exercises, unless it genuinely happens accidentally!

Step 1. Genital Exploration and Stimulation, Focusing on Feelings, but Without Allowing Even the Slightest Trace of an Erection

Use a suitable lubricant, such as warmed-up baby oil. Close your eyes as you explore and manipulate yourself, and **focus on what you are feeling. Immediately** cease genital stimulation if you become aware of **any degree** of penile enlargement! If you have to do this, continue pleasuring some other portion of your body until your penis has **completely** returned to its normal non-erect size. Then, resume genital stimulation. Make sure you try different kinds of touching and stimulation — everything you can think of, although not necessarily in each and every session. Don't restrict yourself exclusively to your penis — also caress and stimulate your testicles, scrotum, upper inner thighs, and the area under your scrotum, in front of your anus. Continue for approximately 15 minutes. If at the end of this time you feel that you would like to continue pleasuring yourself until you ejaculate, **do not do so!** It is **very** important that you do **not** have an orgasm at the end of this exercise! If you are very turned on, try the cold shower remedy!

If you get any feeling that ejaculation is not far away, **immediately** cease genital stimulation, as above. **Do not resume genital**

manipulation until any such feeling has completely and absolutely vanished! Of course, if inadvertently you do ejaculate, it can't be helped, although you will then terminate the exercise for that occasion.

Repeat this first step on as many separate occasions as it takes for you to know that you have explored every kind of touching and stimulation you can think of, on each and every portion of your genital area, while focusing on your sensations. No matter what, **never** move to the next step, until this first one has been practised on at least 6 separate occasions. Usually, you will need more practice than this!

Step 2. *Genital Stimulation, Focusing on Feelings, Until a Degree of Penile Expansion has been Achieved*

This is done exactly as in step 1, but now you will use the kinds of penile manipulation which you have learned are most stimulating. Don't forget the non-genital 'warm-up'! **Do not, under any circumstances, actively try to make your penis enlarge!** Simply stimulate yourself, focus on your genital feelings, and keep all other thoughts out of your mind, using thought stopping if necessary. Allow your penis to do whatever it wants to do! As soon as you become aware that it has begun to enlarge a little, **immediately** stop stimulating it, and continue stroking and caressing your inner thighs and lower abdomen. When it has shrunk back to its normal resting size, begin stimulating again until it expands **just a little,** then change over to non-penile caressing until it goes down completely. Continue thus for 20 minutes, then stop **without** giving yourself an orgasm at the end — this prohibition is **crucially** important!

When you repeat this exercise in the next practice session, continue stimulating yourself until your penis has enlarged **just a little more** than it did in the last exercise session.

When you repeat this exercise in your next practice period, continue until it has expanded **just a little more** than you permitted in the previous session. Continue, slowly progressing, until after perhaps a dozen separate practice periods, you will be continuing stimulation until your penis has been allowed to grow to a size that would probably be adequate for vaginal penetration, **even though it may not have become fully hard!**

As in the first step, should you get **any** sensation that ejaculation is not far away, **immediately** cease genital stimulation, and do not resume it, until any such feeling has **completely and absolutely vanished.** If you inadvertently ejaculate, it can't be helped, simply terminate the exercise for that occasion.

Remember

1. Follow the instructions **exactly** as I have spelt them out!
2. Always get in the correct frame of mind first, and **make sure you are completely relaxed and remain that way.** Use a non-genital 'warm-up'!
3. At all times, focus on your physical genital sensations.
4. Always lubricate your penis, scrotum, lower abdomen and inner thighs.
5. Never **try** to **make** your penis enlarge — let it do whatever it fancies on any particular occasion.
6. With repeated practice in different sessions, allow your penis to expand only **just a little more** than you permitted in the previous session.
7. Make haste slowly! If you finish this exercise in fewer than a dozen separate sessions, you are going too fast. **Often many more** than 12 sessions are required to properly master this sequence!

Possible Problems

The main one is that your penis might be behaving stubbornly, refusing to enlarge, or expanding a little, but then no more. If this occurs, check to make sure you have obeyed all my rules and instructions, **to the letter!** If you haven't, get your conditions right, and start all over again from the beginning, now doing this procedure **exactly** correctly! If you have in fact done it **absolutely correctly,** cut your losses and stop the exercise for this occasion. The next time you do it, first get your conditions right, then experiment with the following suggestions:

1. While doing the exercise, use both hands on your penis, instead of just one. With your clumsy hand (left for most of us), steady your penis at its base, and at the same time, hold all the loose skin firmly down at the base, so it cannot move up and down over the penis. If it helps, with this same hand, you can gently compress the base of the penis, acting a bit like a tourniquet, to stop blood flowing out too quickly. Then, with your other hand, **vigorously stimulate** your lubricated penis. Concentrate on the region around the head and upper shaft, as for most of us, this is the area of maximum sensitivity. Even though you are now stimulating yourself vigorously, scrupulously avoid **trying** to **make** your penis enlarge! As always, it has a mind of its own, and you simply must let it do whatever it chooses on each particular occasion!

2. Some men report that this exercise is a lot easier to do when they are soaking in a warm (not hot) bath. This is physically relaxing, and may better suit your penis.

   If a fair trial of these extra suggestions does not help over several sessions, simply skip this second step, and move on to step 3.

Step 3. Genital Stimulation, Focusing on Feelings and a Sexual Fantasy, but Without Permitting Penile Expansion

This is done similarly to step 1 (self-stimulation, focusing on feelings but **with even the slightest degree of penile enlargement prohibited),** except that now as you manipulate yourself, you are to imagine one of the sexual fantasies you have been practising (appendix 7). **Remember, it takes some considerable practice to self-stimulate, focus on feelings, and lose yourself in a fantasy.** Simply do your best, and in a dozen 15-minute practice sessions or so, you will have got the hang of it. Continue practising until you are **fully confident** that you can **easily** do it. If during step 3 your penis begins to expand, continue with the fantasy, but change to caressing and stimulating other skin areas nearby, until it has **completely** gone down again.

Deal with any feelings of impending ejaculation as described in step 2.

Step 4. Genital Stimulation, Focusing on Feelings and a Sexual Fantasy, Permitting Gradually Increasing Penile Expansion

This is done exactly as was step 2, but now you will use one of your favourite rehearsed sexual fantasies as well. In the first session you will stop penile stimulation as soon as you get a tiny degree of expansion. In the second session, you will continue until it has expanded just a little more, and so on, until after many separate sessions, you continue until it is standing up to a degree adequate for vaginal penetration.

Deal with any feelings of impending ejaculation as described in step 2.

Do not move on to the joint exercises, until in this last step, you are **fully confident** of your ability to erect to a degree adequate for penetration, without in any way **trying** to do so! Make haste slowly! Curb your impatience!

While you are working through the initial joint exercises, continue practising step 4 by yourself, at least twice weekly, until you commence the joint **erectile** exercises. You can then stop this individual practice.

If on any particular occasion, you encounter difficulties in step 4, because your penis has decided for some reason to be stubborn, follow the procedures suggested in step 2, under 'possible problems'!

Should your penis **persistently** fail to cooperate, **despite** your doing everything exactly as described, and under good conditions, simply cut your losses and cease doing this exercise. **Don't then worry or consider yourself a failure! Remember, not every exercise is right for, or helpful for, every person or every penis!** Progress then to the initial joint exercises.

What Do You Do if You Haven't Got a Cooperative Partner, and Despite Correctly Performing Your Individual Erectile Exercises, You Still Can't Erect Adequately for Penetration?

This is the point at which you should seek professional assistance. You would first get your doctor to meticulously check you out for, and deal with, any physical contributions to your problem. Unless that fixes it, you would then seek expert sex therapy.

If you haven't got a partner, but have successfully completed these individual erectile exercises, **read now** the relevant parts of chapter 12, and appendices 16, 17 and **apply what is suggested there.** Continue practising step 4 at least twice weekly, until you are totally confident of your erectile ability.

Appendix 11

SEXUAL COMMUNICATION EXERCISE

To do this, you will need to buy a suitable book on the techniques of lovemaking. There are many excellent ones on the subject, available from all major booksellers. Purchase one that seems right for you, after browsing through the whole range. Some are a bit highbrow, or hard to read, or boring. Others may be unsuitable for you, for some particular reason. Many find Alex Comfort's *Joy of Sex* excellent, although it assumes that the reader starts off with a fair degree of sexual knowledge and sophistication.

This book is **not** being purchased to provide you with factual information, although virtually every couple practising this exercise learns something new from whatever one they select. **Its primary use** is to help you and your partner learn to communicate easily and comfortably about all aspects of normal lovemaking and sexual expression. Here is how you use your book:

1. Read the first page aloud to your partner. As you do so, either of you are free to interrupt to comment, ask a question and so on. At the end of the page, **together** discuss what has been read. When this has been done, your partner will read the next page to you, in the same way.

2. Put a time limit of 15 minutes on this exercise, which, if possible, should be repeated every day. A little done often is **far** more rewarding than infrequent lengthy sessions.

You will find that as you work through the book, it becomes easier and easier to express your own views and feelings about all the various aspects of lovemaking, in a way that would not have been possible if you had merely discussed lovemaking together without the use of the book. Almost everyone who perseveres with this exercise, which may take many months to complete, reports that they have achieved the following:

1. A much greater awareness of their own individual sexuality, likes, dislikes, preferences, anxieties, fantasies and so on.
2. A greatly increased awareness of their partner's sexuality, needs, wishes, dislikes and preferences.
3. An ability easily and comfortably to discuss **absolutely any** aspect of sexual expression, without shyness or embarrassment.

I think you will find that these benefits will greatly enhance your love-life together, indirectly decrease concerns about performance, and increase arousability and the effectiveness of sexual technique.

Appendix 12

SHARED SENSUALITY EXERCISES

Let it be clearly stated, at the outset, that **this** exercise sequence is probably **the most important single thing** you and your partner can do to resurrect your sex life! How well or otherwise you do this will determine more than anything else the ultimate quality of the sexual relationship you achieve together!

Do yourself a favour — perform these exercises **thoroughly,** and **strictly** according to the instructions, until you have clearly achieved **all** the specific goals!

Step 1

This is a touching exercise, done naked. You **must** have **good conditions** for doing it — privacy, freedom from interruption, a warm room. Additionally, you must not be tired, uptight or preoccupied. If you have difficulty finding half an hour under such conditions, there must be something wrong with your style of living, and your first task together will be to work out how you can get your circumstances right! The commonest problem is getting privacy and having peace of mind when there are young children awake in the house. You may have to farm them out to a friend or relative for a few hours — if you are really motivated to overcome your problem, **you will somehow find a way!** Remember to take your phone off the hook!

Undress each other until you are totally naked. Then, flip a coin, or in some other democratic way, decide who will be the toucher to start with. The partner to be touched lies naked on the bed, face up or face down. The room light should be on. The toucher has the job of pleasurably touching the partner absolutely anywhere, **but not on the breasts or genitals, which are absolutely forbidden!** The toucher is **not** in any way trying to arouse the partner sexually — the aim is just to produce nice feelings. Should one or other of you get turned on, that is just bad luck, as **under no circumstances is this exercise to be followed by any form of lovemaking or private masturbation!** You are not meant to get aroused, and if you do, you will just have to try a long cold shower or a few hundred push-ups, to get rid of your arousal!

Don't make the mistake of only touching your partner with your hands! You can touch with your nose, lips, tongue, elbow, rump, big toe and so on, and in due course you should try touching with all these, and anything else you can think of! One of the ultimate goals is to have tried every conceivable kind of touching on every part of each other's body.

The person on the receiving end has the job of closing the eyes and giving a non-stop **(literally that — without a pause!)** running commentary on what the touching feels like (in detail), and in what ways it is liked or disliked. The touched person is at liberty to give specific directions, make requests and so on.

After about 15 minutes, you swap places, so that the first toucher becomes the touched. Finish the exercise after about 15 minutes each way. If you don't feel like going for the full time on any particular occasion, stop sooner — for heaven's sake **don't force yourself** to stick it out for the recommended 15 minutes!

A Possible Problem

If you haven't had any sexual contact with your partner for a while, the idea of suddenly being naked together with the light on may be a bit embarrassing or even scarey. You need to know that **most** couples actually feel a bit stupid or embarrassed the first time, perhaps because the whole performance is contrived and novel rather than

spontaneous and familiar. It is perfectly all right to start off in a rather
less embarrassing way if you feel like it! You might, for example,
do it initially in the dark, or with night attire or underwear on,
gradually progressing to complete nakedness with the light on.

Some Variations

You may be interested to do the exercise when the room is
illuminated by a red light, or by candles. You will probably find that
your bodies then look more sensual, and you may feel more comfortable when the worst of what ageing has done to you is rather less
conspicuous!

In at least several sessions you should try the exercise with the
aid of some body lotion or massage oil — you will find this a different,
very sensual experience. If you are worried about messing up your
sheets, use a couple of coloured towels underneath you.

Particularly if you find yourselves a little light on ideas about
different kinds of sensual, non-sexual touching, you might care to
systematically work through the suggestions in a book on sensual
massage — see the reading list in appendix 18.

Goals to be Achieved Before You Move on to the Second Step

1. You should have tried every kind of touching you can think of
   on every part of each other's body, except for the breasts and
   genitals.
2. You should feel **completely** relaxed during the exercise, and
   actually enjoy the experience.
3. You should have mastered the art of non-stop talking about what
   you are feeling and how you like it or dislike it.
4. You should be very comfortable giving each other instructions
   as to exactly what you would like done to you.

I have **never** met any couple who have genuinely achieved
these goals in fewer than 6 half-hour sessions, and I can tell you
from considerable experience that most couples require **many more**

than these 6 sessions to achieve their goals! **Make haste slowly — these particular exercises are crucially important!**

You may think all this sounds very simple (and it is!) and wonder how it could be so important. Suffice it to say that in this apparently simple exercise there are actually a large number of important things happening, which are not obvious at first.

It is a sad fact that for many people, doing this exercise is the first opportunity they have had in their whole life to relate physically, naked, without any need to perform or achieve some particular goal!

Step 2

When you can **honestly** say that you have achieved **all** the goals of the first part of these exercises, you are ready for the next step. This is essentially the same as the first one, except that the focus of attention is exclusively on the breasts (both male and female) and genitals — i.e. the parts of the body which were forbidden in the first exercise.

Even though frankly sexual parts of your bodies are now going to be touched, you are not meant to get turned on or aroused! Getting aroused is actually a nuisance because it distracts you from really learning as much as you can about yourself and your partner. If you do become aroused, that is just bad luck, as there is no lovemaking or masturbation at the end! Try the cold shower treatment or something similar! **If you start to get even a bit of an erection, stop genital touching immediately** and have a cuddle until your penis goes down completely. **Under no circumstances** are you to allow yourself to achieve any penile enlargement in this exercise!

When exploring and fondling your female partner's genital area, you simply **must** use some form of lubricant, or you will cause her discomfort. If you don't have a pleasantly perfumed body lotion or massage oil, you can use warmed-up baby oil!

Because the breast and genital areas are relatively small, many people make the mistake of thinking that it won't take long to fully explore them. Small they may be, but you need to examine them in meticulous detail! You might, for example, be seeing what one index finger, rubbing gently on one square centimetre of one inner lip, feels like for your partner. You aim to systematically explore the sensate (feeling) potential of every little nook and cranny, every area of skin. It will take you at least 6 half-hour sessions, and probably many more, to achieve the goals of step 2, which are the same as the goals of step 1.

Remember: under no circumstances are you to engage in any form of lovemaking, or to masturbate, after either step of this exercise! You ignore this advice at your own peril!

Appendix 13

JOINT ERECTILE EXERCISES

Before you start these, you **must** have thoroughly worked through the individual erectile exercises, described in appendix 10, **and** the shared sensuality exercises, as described in appendix 12.

Before you go any further, re-read appendix 10, as you will now be doing something very similar together. **Note carefully the general rules!**

Most couples find that the most comfortable position for the initial joint erectile exercises, is that depicted in figure 8. Your partner, who is naked, sits upright in bed, with her back supported by pillows placed against the bed-head or wall. Her legs are reasonably straight, and fairly wide apart. You lie naked on your back in the opposite direction, your head facing the other end of the bed. You have your legs over her thighs, so that your genital area is quite comfortably within her reach, close to her own genitals.

Step 1.   Genital Stimulation, with You Focusing on Your Physical Feelings, with Your Eyes Closed, but Without Allowing Yourself to Get Even the Slightest Trace of an Erection

The instructions are generally as for appendix 10, step 1, except that your partner is now providing the stimulation. Because you have already done the shared sensuality exercises together, your partner

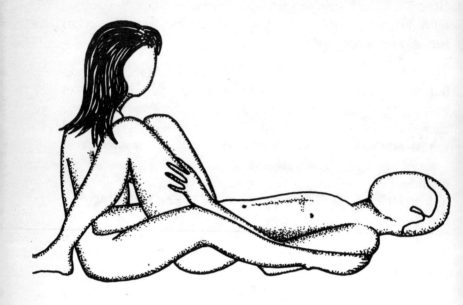

*Fig. 8 The most comfortable position for the initial shared
erection exercises*

is not required to **explore** your genitals, as you were when you did
it by yourself. She is trying to give you arousing stimulation, but
without you allowing any degree of penile enlargement.

Deal with any feelings of impending ejaculation, by **immediately
ceasing genital stimulation,** until such feelings have **completely**
disappeared. Should you **inadvertently ejaculate,** it can't be
helped — simply stop the exercise at that point, until next time.

**Remember: unless it genuinely happens accidentally, there
must be no orgasm/ejaculation during or at the end of this or
the subsequent exercises!**

After at least 6 practice sessions, and then only when you are totally
confident that in this exercise you can easily focus on your physical
genital sensations, and remain completely relaxed, move on to the
next step.

Step 2.   Genital Stimulation, Focusing on Feelings, with Your Eyes Closed, Until a Degree of Penile Expansion has Been Achieved

The directions are essentially the same as in step 2, appendix 10, but with your partner providing the stimulation. Re-read the instructions there very carefully, together. Remember, under no circumstances are you in any way to **try** to make your penis enlarge! Let it do whatever it chooses on any particular occasion!

Continue this step in repeated sessions until you are **totally** confident that in this exercise your penis will consistently enlarge to a degree that would be suitable for vaginal penetration, then move on.

If you have any difficulties, follow the suggestions described under 'Possible Problems' in the individual erectile exercises, with your partner doing whatever previously you were to do yourself. If these suggestions do not help, simply skip this second step and move on to step 3.

Step 3.   Partner Stimulation of Penis, Without any Degree of Penis Enlargement Permitted, While You Use a Sexual Fantasy and Continue to Focus on Your Genital Feelings

Follow the directions for step 3, appendix 10. When you find it easy to do what is required, progress to the next step.

Step 4.   Partner Stimulation of Penis, While You Use a Sexual Fantasy and Focus on Genital Feelings, but with Progressively Increasing Penile Expansion Permitted

See step 4, appendix 10. Repeat this until you are **totally** confident that you can do what is required, i.e. consistently erect to a degree adequate for vaginal penetration.

If you have any difficulties, again follow the suggestions described under 'Possible Problems', in the individual erectile exercises, with your partner doing what previously you were to do yourself. If these do not help, simply skip this fourth step, and move on to step 5.

Step 5.   Vaginal Insertion of Your Totally Limp Penis

This is a procedure which is technically described by the singularly unattractive phrase, 'vaginal stuffing'! You do this in a special position, known as the 'scissors' position. You will need to master this before you can begin this step. Practise getting into the scissors a few times with your clothes still on — it is not difficult, but it does take a bit of practice to achieve it, without in any way having to think about what you are doing.

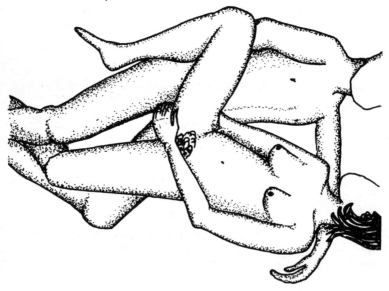

Fig. 9 The so-called 'scissors' position for use in the shared erection exercises

Scissors Position (see figure 9)

Your partner lies flat on her back on the bed, with her knees drawn up, so that the angle between her thighs and calves is about 45 degrees. You then lie on your **left** side, underneath her legs, at right angles to her body, facing towards her. Your bodies will now form a cross, with your genitals nearly touching. Next, move around towards her, so that you can put your left arm around her. It may help if as you do this, she moves over **just a little** towards her left side. Next, intertwine your legs so that they are arranged with your left leg on the bottom, against the bed. Her left leg will now be sandwiched between your two legs, and her right leg will be on top, over your right hip, with her right heel on or near the bed. It sounds complicated, but it really is **extremely simple** to achieve, and this is one of, if not the, most relaxed and comfortable intercourse positions you will ever find!

How to Perform Step 5

Get your partner to lubricate your penis **and** her genitals and hands, with some warmed baby oil, while you are in the scissors position with your limp penis almost directly touching her vagina. **Use plenty of lubricant!** If you have **even the slightest trace of an erection,** this is a nuisance, and you will just have to wait until it decides to go down! Your partner then practises tucking your limp penis into her vagina, using both hands. She might use the fingers of her left (clumsy) hand to spread her vaginal lips and open her vaginal entrance, while the fingers of her right (good) hand tuck the head of the penis in. Once it is in, both hands can be used to feed in as much of the shaft as possible. It often helps if she contracts and relaxes her vaginal (pelvic) muscles during the tucking-in process.

It usually requires quite a deal of practice to master this skill, but make a fun thing of your efforts, and if it seems too difficult the first time, give up before you get frustrated, and try again later on. Remember, **your penis must be completely limp!** It is of course possible, in fact much easier, to tuck in a semi-erect penis, but this exercise is **only** concerned with learning to tuck in a **completely limp penis.**

If your partner has long finger nails, she may have to trim them or she could accidentally hurt your penis while learning to tuck it in. **When she is an expert, she can do the job even with long nails!**

When your limp penis has been successfully inserted (tucked) into your partner's vagina, leave it there for about a minute, without making any movement, then withdraw it, and repeat the insertion process some half-dozen times in that practice session. Repeat step 5 however many times it takes until you are **both** confident that insertion of your limp penis can be quickly and easily achieved in the scissors position.

Throughout this exercise, you are to remain **totally passive!** You are **not** to try to help with the tucking-in process in any way! Your only contribution is to provide a completely limp penis! Keep your eyes closed, and just concentrate on whatever feelings you experience in your penis, pleasant or otherwise, as your partner gets the hang of this manoeuvre.

If for some reason, after plenty of practice, you still find penetration with a limp penis in this position difficult, **then** you can assist your partner in the following way: In the scissors position, put your right thumb and forefinger tightly around the base of your penis, to act like an incomplete tourniquet. This will artificially stiffen the end of your penis, making it easier for your partner to insert it.

If during this exercise, you get **any** feelings that ejaculation is not far away, **immediately** ask your partner to stop what she is doing, until these sensations have **completely** disappeared. If however you do inadvertently ejaculate, **carry on with the exercise as if you had not!**

Step 6. Vaginal Penetration in the Scissors Position with a Limp Penis, with Limited Thrusting, Still with a Limp Penis

This is done as in the previous step, but now you must learn to 'thrust' without an erection. To enable this, your partner **must** hold your penis between the index and middle fingers of her right hand (left, if it happens to be more comfortable), to prevent it slipping out, **and** to compress it to produce a partial tourniquet-like effect.

You may need to use your right thumb and forefinger, like a tourniquet, as well.

It may help considerably if as you 'thrust' **in,** your partner deliberately **relaxes** her vaginal (pelvic) muscles, then **contracts** them as you move **out.** For her to be able to do this really effectively, and automatically, she will need regularly to practise the pelvic muscle exercise (appendix 6).

Be prepared to have to put in quite a bit of practice to get the hang of limited thrusting without an erection.

If, while you are performing this step, you begin to erect, this is a nuisance, and you will just have to stop until it goes down again!

When, in one practice run, it is obvious that you could quite easily continue limited thrusting with a limp penis, more or less as long as you wished, stop, disconnect, and have a rest before recommencing the same exercise. Repeat 6 times in each practice session.

If at any stage you feel that ejaculation is not too far away, **immediately** stop whatever you are doing, and wait until this sensation of impending ejaculation has **completely disappeared.** Then, resume where you left off. Should you accidentally ejaculate, it can't be helped — simply carry on with the exercise.

Occasionally, for one reason or another, a couple find stuffing and/or movement with a limp penis just too difficult to achieve. If this applies to you, after you have done the best you can, simply quit. **Do not feel that you have then failed! Remember that not every procedure is right for every couple or every penis!**

The Next Step

Exactly what you do now, depends upon whether or not your partner can manipulate you to an erection which would be adequate for 'unassisted' vaginal penetration. This means penetration without her having to use any of the special skills involved in vaginal stuffing.

If you have successfully completed Step 4 of these joint erectile exercises, you can now be manipulated to an erection adequate for normal vaginal penetration. You then progress through the remaining steps, described below.

If you have not been able to satisfactorily complete step 4, **do
not attempt these remaining steps!**

Step 7.   Vaginal Penetration in the 'Female Superior' Position, Without any Movement Permitted After Entry, Then Allowing the Penis to go Completely Limp Inside the Vagina

What is the Female Superior Position?

This is illustrated in figure 10. You lie naked, flat on your back, legs
out straight and close together. Your naked partner kneels astride
you, taking her weight on her legs and feet, which are placed on
either side of your body. She partially sits on your thighs, facing you,
with the upper part of her body just a little forward from being

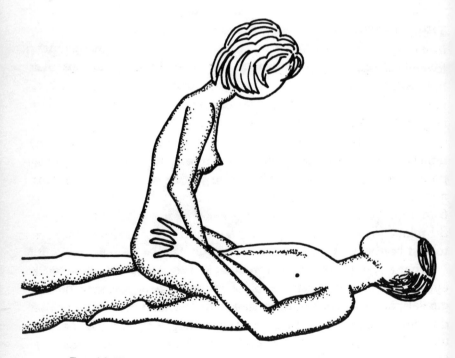

*Fig. 10 The female superior position for use in the shared
erection exercises*

perpendicular to you. Your penis and her genitals will be very close to each other.

How to Perform Step 7

In this position, your partner **generously** lubricates your penis and her genitals, using baby oil or a massage oil.

She then stimulates your penis with both hands, until it is hard enough for penetration. This should be easy, as you have already mastered this skill in step 4, described above. She then leans forward slightly, spreads her vaginal lips with the fingers of her clumsy (left) hand, and uses her good (right) hand to guide your penis in. It may be best if her good hand operates from behind her buttocks, rather than from the front.

If there is any difficulty with insertion, because the penis is not quite hard enough, your partner can try the following modification:

She shifts her weight to the left side of her body and her left leg. Then, she brings her right leg forward, so that the sole of her right foot rests firmly on the bed. She can now more easily use both hands to feed your penis in. After insertion has been achieved, she resumes the normal female superior position. If in the process of insertion your erection goes down, commence this step again from the beginning.

When you are inside her, neither of you move, and you both wait until your penis has **fully** gone down, inside her vagina. Then, your partner dismounts and lies down for a minute or so to rest her legs and back, before repeating the whole process. You should aim for 6 mounts in each practice session, which will probably take 20 to 30 minutes, depending on how much time your partner chooses to rest between mounts.

What are you doing, while all this is going on? You have your eyes closed, you concentrate on the feelings you experience in your genitals, and lose yourself in a pleasing sexual fantasy. You otherwise do nothing but provide a penis. If it arouses you to fondle your partner while she is doing her thing, **and** if she is in agreement, feel free to go ahead, but keep your eyes closed, and continue to focus on your feelings and a fantasy.

If at any stage, you experience feelings that you might soon ejaculate, **immediately stop whatever is being done, and wait until these feelings have completely gone away.** Then, resume from the beginning. Should you inadvertently ejaculate, it can't be helped. Simply finish the exercise at that point, until your next practice session.

When you are **completely confident** that in this position you can **repeatedly** erect adequately for penetration, let it go down inside her vagina, and again erect adequately for penetration, you are ready to move onto the next step.

Step 8. Vaginal Penetration in the Female Superior Position, with You, but not Your Partner, Moving Slowly After Entry

This is done exactly as in step 7, but after your partner has inserted your penis, you begin to move it slowly in and out. She does not move at all. You are **not** trying to reach an orgasm or in any way get her aroused! While you are slowly moving in and out, you will have your eyes closed, you will be focusing on your genital feelings, and you will be fantasizing. As previously, fondling your partner is an optional extra. **When it is obvious that you could continue moving like this more or less as long as you wanted, still keeping whatever degree of erection you started with, stop moving and let your partner dismount,** to give her a rest. Repeat the sequence 6 times in each practice session.

Handle any feelings of impending ejaculation as in step 7.

Continue this step in subsequent sessions, until you are completely confident that you can get your penis in, move slowly, keep it as expanded as it was to start with, not slip out, and repeat this sequence without any difficulty. Then and only then, are you ready to move onto the next step.

Step 9. Vaginal Penetration in the Female Superior Position, with You Both Moving Slowly After Entry

This is done exactly as in step 8, except that now your partner also moves slowly. You keep going until it is obvious that you could continue this more or less as long as you wanted, still keeping whatever degree of erection you started with. Then stop to give your partner a rest, before repeating the exercise.

You are ready for the final step when you are totally confident of your ability repeatedly to perform this procedure in a single practice session, without any difficulty.

Deal with any feelings of impending ejaculation as in step 7.

Step 10. Vaginal Penetration in the Scissors Position, with You Both Moving Slowly After Entry

This is done exactly as was step 9, but once again using the scissors position.

When you are totally convinced that you can perform this procedure repeatedly, in a single practice session, without any difficulty, you should be very confident of your ability to erect adequately for intercourse!

Now, and only now, is the complete prohibition on any attempt at vaginal penetration during lovemaking lifted! From now on, when you feel like making love, if you wish, you can have intercourse. Of course, sometimes you won't feel like intercourse, and with your new attitude to lovemaking, you will just enjoy yourselves in whatever way suits the mood you are both in. **However, for a while, follow carefully the suggestions in appendix 14!**

What Do You Do If, In Spite of Performing the Joint Erectile Exercises Absolutely Correctly, You Still Can't Erect Adequately for Normal Vaginal Penetration?

This is the point at which you should seek professional assistance. You would first get your doctor meticulously to check you out for, and deal with, any physical contributions to your problem. Unless that fixes it, you would then seek expert therapy.

While all this is being enacted, unless you are instructed otherwise, practise insertion and thrusting without an erection, in the scissors position only, until you have both got this down to a really fine art. Then, do the same thing again, repeatedly, but now using a sexual fantasy during the exercise. If your partner is agreeable, you can now **also** fondle her. Remember to focus on your genital feelings, as well as the fantasy.

When you can **easily** do all this, the previous prohibition on any attempt at vaginal penetration during spontaneous lovemaking could be removed, and when you make love, you could have intercourse with a limp penis, **if you wish! However, use only the scissors position!** You will naturally have to employ the skills you have learned to enable you to penetrate and 'thrust' without an erection.

If you find it difficult to ejaculate inside the vagina with a limp penis, you may have to be manipulated to orgasm outside the vagina, when intercourse is no longer desired. You will probably also need to bring your partner to orgasm by hand stimulation.

Often, you will find that once you know that you can actually have a form of intercourse without an erection, any pressure on getting one disappears. You then worry progressively less, and your maximum erection may steadily increase. Meticulously and thoroughly do everything else suggested in the book, so you have as much going for you as possible.

What Do You Do If Expert Assistance Fails to Restore Adequate Potency?

You might get a second independent expert opinion, before deciding that your problem is insoluble. Should you be forced to this conclusion, **do not despair!** Reflect with your partner on your options (see chapter 12), and pursue whichever course of action seems best for you both.

Notes for Women on the Joint Erectile Exercises

No one has **any** illusions that there is any pleasure for you in these exercises! They represent something that you are doing to help your partner, because you care about him, and want to assist. Your uncomplaining, patient cooperation and persistence will however be well rewarded for the following reasons:

a. When the erection problem has been overcome, you personally will have more sexual options during lovemaking.

b. You will find that your cooperation brings you much closer together as a couple, strengthening your relationship and the bond between you.

c. You will find that your partner will not forget what you have done for him! The appreciation of an impotent man, assisted to cure by his partner, **never dies!** Like the proverbial elephant, an ex-impotent man does not forget her help! This will enrich your own life in all sorts of ways.

Some final comments

The most frequent error that women make in pursuing this exercise sequence, is in being **too gentle** when they stimulate the penis by hand. Unlike a woman's genitals, which are very delicate and require extremely careful handling, penises are pretty tough customers which have survived all sorts of rough handling, such as being dragged up and down football fields, being caught in barbed-wire fences, zippers and the like! **In the exercises, hand-stimulate your partner's penis vigorously!** You can't hurt him, as long as you use adequate lubrication! Re-read the section in chapter 12, on ejaculating without an erection, for some extra hints on effective penile stimulation. Remember that your partner is the leading world expert on the best and most arousing way to stimulate his penis, **so don't hesitate to ask him to give you a few tips, perhaps even to show you the most effective way of manipulating him!**

Appendix 14

HINTS ABOUT LOVEMAKING WHEN INTERCOURSE IS ONCE AGAIN PERMITTED

When you have overcome your problem through the exercises, intercourse during lovemaking is once again allowed. However, you will find that **even though** you are now actually able to achieve vaginal penetration and thrusting virtually whenever you wish, it will take **many months** before you approach lovemaking feeling **totally confident** of your ability to do so! In other words, it will be a long time before you make love, without the **slightest thought** that perhaps your penis won't do the right thing by you! This delay is **absolutely normal!**

Until you have reached the stage where you approach lovemaking joyously, without **any** thoughts about erection difficulties, even though your penis is consistently doing the right thing, you should:

1. Mainly use the scissors position for intercourse. This is because it is usually the most relaxed and comfortable position of all, and in it your partner can most easily help with any minor difficulties, by: tucking ('stuffing') you in; using her pelvic (vaginal) muscles; using her good hand around the base of your penis to give you extra stimulation, or to act as a gentle tourniquet.

    As an important aside, this is also a wonderful position for your partner, as she does not feel 'crowded' or pinned down, can move freely as she wishes, and can have you comfortably stimulate her breasts and clitoris **as** you thrust into her.

2. Continue to practise step 2 from appendix 13, once a week, as an exercise unrelated to lovemaking, and with **no** orgasm allowed! Start off right from the beginning, when you get around to repeating this step after resuming intercourse in lovemaking.

3. Agree together that every third time you make love, vaginal penetration will not occur under any circumstances! You will then of course use non-intercourse techniques to satisfy each other.

Remember that sooner or later, virtually **every man** on this planet won't erect adequately on some particular occasion, when he would wish to! This is usually because he has ignored his personal 'conditions'! It is not a matter of **will** you **ever** again have difficulty getting or keeping an erection, but a simple question of how long it will be until this once again occurs! Remember, **it is the same for every other man!** That's just the way it is — **it is normal, and inevitable,** and you simply can't expect to be better than normal! When next your penis chooses to go against your wishes during lovemaking, do the following:

1. Laugh **out loud,** to yourself and your partner, at its antics! For example, you might jokingly say something like this: 'Poor old Percy has gone on strike! Perhaps I haven't been feeding him well enough!'

2. Then, say something like this: 'Who cares, we'll still have a wonderful time, and we might even try some special goodies!'

3. **Never ever, under any circumstances, apologize or say you are sorry!** There is **nothing** to apologize for! You are not doing something deliberately to deprive her of anything! Furthermore, there is absolutely no logical reason why you should in any way put yourself down (which an apology often involves), for something which happens normally to **all** men from time to time!

4. Press on with lovemaking, concentrating on giving and receiving as much pleasure as possible, including orgasm if that is desired.

5. **Never work at erecting, and don't allow your partner to keep trying to get you up! As soon as** you notice that your penis probably isn't interested in cooperating on this particular occasion, do what I have suggested above, and **completely give up** on the idea of an erection for the rest of this lovemaking session! **Don't make the mistake of coming back later on and having another go at persuading your penis to change its mind!**

6. During and after that lovemaking session, and especially just before and during the next session, do not allow yourself to have **even one single thought about erections!** Use thought stopping against any such thoughts, **with a vengeance!** Remember, logically, there truly is **nothing to worry about!** However, if you let your mind think about erections, you will (irrationally) begin to worry, and this will then probably interfere with your penis' ability to be cooperative next time you want it to stand up!

7. Agree with your partner in advance that the next time you make love together, there will be **absolutely no attempt** at vaginal penetration, even if you have a perfect erection! This will take the pressure off your penis and help to stop you worrying.

Appendix 15

SUGGESTIONS FOR EXERCISES TO OVERCOME THE EFFECTS OF DESTRUCTIVE SEXUAL MYTHS

Over and above the specific procedures listed in chapter 5, you can adapt some of the 'doing' exercises described in appendix 1, to help you overcome the effects of some particularly personally destructive myth.

You can, for example, as an exercise, **deliberately** engage in some form of sexual behaviour, with the proviso that whatever you have previously believed should occur, **must under no circumstances be allowed to occur!** For example, if you are working to overcome the destructive effects of the myth that males must always be active during sex, make a deal with your partner that as an exercise, sexual contact will occur where she will be responsible for absolutely everything. You will remain totally passive, quite literally doing nothing until and unless you are given a firm instruction to do something to or for her.

Self-monitoring (appendix 1, exercise 3) is very useful in tackling almost any myth (or automatic illogical way of thinking) that you wish to overcome. However, **only** use it against **one** myth at a time! If you are using it against a couple of sexual myths simultaneously, you will make the technique less effective.

Discussing in detail with your partner your **irrational feelings** or emotions associated with and based on a myth, can be very helpful, as described in appendix 1, exercise 4. Likewise, teaching and persuading others that the myth is truly absurd (appendix 1, exercise 6), is a powerful procedure for helping yourself.

Talking to the myth like a naughty child is often effective (appendix 1, exercise 7), as is the 'exaggerated worrying out loud' about the present and future implications for you of the myth being true (appendix 1, exercise 8).

The Premack technique and autosuggestion are widely applicable and helpful, but as with self-monitoring, **only use them against one particular myth at a time!** Don't forget to re-write the myth in **logical, positive terms** when you use these 2 procedures.

Appendix 16

SOME HINTS ON THE FIRST TIME WITH A NEW PARTNER

Most men and women feel at least some anxiety the first time they have sex with a new partner, unless perhaps it is a purely commercial transaction. The reasons for this are numerous, but in essence we tend to feel somewhat insecure in this situation, because we are then potentially so emotionally vulnerable. Of course, some people go to great lengths to try to conceal their anxiety, but the astute observer can still often pick it up!

The Basic Rule

Never under any circumstances get into a sexual situation with a new partner, unless **most** of your personal conditions for being sexually responsive are met! Remember the message of chapter 6!
   Especially relevant are the following:
   1. **Don't** get involved in sexual contact **unless you genuinely feel sexually interested!**
   2. **Don't** get into a sexual situation if you are **in any way** tense, anxious, angry, guilty and so on!

Some Important Points

   1. First, get to know your partner over a number of social meetings, to get comfortable with her, and to determine if **you really want to have sex with her.**

2. Remember, there is no law that says you **have** to have sex just because you have an opportunity to do so, or because you are with a partner who wants to. If you don't feel comfortable, or don't feel like sex, you could say something like this: 'It probably sounds quaint, but making love is something special to me, and as much as you turn me on, I choose to wait until I know you better — it will be much more enjoyable for both of us then'. Far from causing your partner to think there is something wrong with you, she will **respect** you all the more for this approach.

3. You don't have to 'go all the way', first up! You will probably find yourself feeling much more comfortable if you, as it were, wade in gradually, in stages! You could, for example, start with a simple massage for the first few times, then progress to deliberate breast and genital stroking and so on. You might perhaps say something like this: 'I guess I'm old fashioned, but intercourse is something really special for me, and I'd like to know you better in every way before we become completely intimate — we'll both enjoy it so much more then'.

4. A neat, effective way of decreasing your anxiety, is to **admit to being anxious!** Try to express it in a light-hearted manner, for example, by saying something like this: 'It is totally ridiculous, since I feel extremely close to you and very much want to make love with you, but I feel a little anxious — isn't it stupid!'. **By admitting it, you largely overcome it!** Often enough, your partner will have a laugh, and confess to being anxious also, in which case you can both relax, because there is no longer any need to pretend!

5. Remember what I have said about 'levelling', in chapter 12!

Appendix 17

SOME SEXUAL 'BAD HABITS' TO BE AVOIDED OR OVERCOME

Strictly speaking, some of these issues are very largely beyond the immediate subject of this book, but I have chosen to include a brief section on bad habits. Why? Firstly, some of what I have to say will be a useful revision of issues I have raised earlier. Secondly, having shown you how to revamp your sex life by overcoming impotence as an issue in your lovemaking, I would hate to think that you ran the risk of getting less out of sexual relating than you could, merely because I didn't remind you of a few simple facts!

The following bad habits are offered in no particular order, and with minimal elaboration. A little thought should enable you to see what is wrong!

1. Ignoring your 'conditions' for being sexually interested and responsive! This of course applies to **both** you and your partner, and for the pair of you, will become progressively more important as you grow older.
2. Sameness! Do you always make love basically the same way? Do you usually do it at approximately the same time, in the same place? Would you enjoy your favourite food if all you ate, day in, day out, was the same food at the same time, in the same place?
3. Always leaving lovemaking until bedtime! You can't expect to

be creative, sensitive, intuitive, active and sensuous when you are tired at the end of a long day!

4. Fondling the breasts and genitals too quickly after starting, neglecting cuddling together, slow kissing, and caressing other parts of the body!

5. The male doing the inserting of the penis — it should **always** be the woman's job!

6. Failing to talk during lovemaking! You should be conveying endearments, and even more importantly, requests, information and feedback about your wishes and needs.

7. Talking about unrelated events during lovemaking! Your partner gets a very clear message that your mind is elsewhere, which is a real slap-in-the-face for someone who is trying to express their love for you!

8. Being preoccupied with other issues during lovemaking! If you can't devote yourself mentally to what you are experiencing and sharing, what on earth are you doing making love? This is much more than simple bad manners — it is **stupidity** of a very hurtful kind, and frankly **insulting** to your partner!

9. Habitually not having enough time for proper lovemaking! Are you always or often making love, as it were, with one eye on a mental clock?

10. Putting pressure on your partner to have an orgasm! Lovemaking has got **nothing** to do with performance or pressure! Orgasms are **not** in any way essential!

11. Wearing offputting clothing (or even worse) during lovemaking! For example, don't expect your penis to be interested in standing to attention, if your partner has her hair in curlers and a face-mask on, or if she is wearing a dreary nightgown only really fit for polishing the floor! You yourself might shave, and dress up for bed, to present yourself as best possible!

12. Making love when you are smelly!

13. Making love with unclean genitals!

14. Never having an orgasm other than inside the vagina, or for women, one produced by penile thrusting!

15. Never having a non-sexual break during lovemaking! If once you start sexual contact, it **must** relentlessly proceed until

intercourse has been achieved and finished, **you are missing out** on the joys of stop-start lovemaking! This does not mean that you should dive out of bed and mow the lawn between oral-genital stimulation and intercourse, but it does mean that sometimes after arousing each other to a degree, you might just talk, have a laugh, cuddle, enjoy some music and so on, before again commencing sexual stimulation. Who wants to rush through a fabulous 4-course meal without a break between dishes! Stop to enjoy the atmosphere and whet the appetite a little, so that the experience can be as pleasurable as possible!

16. Ceasing all physical and verbal expressions of affection as soon as intercourse ceases! In old-fashioned language, **don't forget the 'afterplay'!**

17. Always having the light **off** when you make love!

18. Hopping out of bed to wash your genitals immediately after intercourse. If you still think sex is dirty, you have a lot of growing up to do!

19. Only showing your partner affection when you want sexual contact!

20. Never engaging in pleasurable physical contact with your partner's sexual organs, except when you intend to carry through and have intercourse! Playful, gentle, loving genital and breast stimulation should be part and parcel of daily affectionate body contact!

Isn't it easy to slip into some bad habits without really realizing that it is happening?

Appendix 18

RECOMMENDED READING

Sexual Myths, Conditions for Being Sexually Responsive

Bernie Zilbergeld: *Men and Sex* (Fontana, 1980). The American edition is titled *Male Sexuality*, and was published by Little, Brown & Company, Boston, 1978

Attitude Change

Arnold Lazarus and Allen Fay: *I Can if I Want to* (New York, 1977)
Albert Ellis and Robert Harper: *A New Guide to Rational Living* (Wilshire Book Company, Hollywood, U.S.A. 1975)

Shared Sensuality Exercises

Gordon Inkeles and Murray Todris: *The Art of Sensual Massage* (Unwin Hyman, 1984)
Gordon Inkeles: *New Massage* (Unwin Hyman, 1984)

Sexual Fantasy

Nancy Friday: *My Secret Garden* (Quartet, 1979)
Nancy Friday: *Forbidden Flowers* (New York, 1982)
Nancy Friday: *Men in Love* (Arrow Books, 1981)

The first two are on female fantasies, and the third is about male fantasies. **All** are worth reading by men.

Sexual Communication Exercise, Lovemaking Techniques

Alex Comfort: *The Joy of Sex* (Quartet Books, London 1976)

You should be able to borrow these books from any sizable library, even if it has to get them in for you. Alternatively, you could purchase them from any major bookseller, although they might have to be specially ordered for you.

Appendix 19

A SIMPLE DESCRIPTION OF SOME TECHNICAL TERMS AS USED IN THIS BOOK

Antidepressant   A drug useful in overcoming a depressive illness.

Anus   The exit of the bowel under the buttocks.

Artery   A tube taking fresh blood to a part of the body.

Atherosclerosis   A common degenerative disease of arteries causing them to become narrower in places.

Autosuggestion   Giving oneself suggestions while in a relaxed state.

Buck's Fascia   A sheath of fibrous tissue holding the 3 cylinders of the penis together.

Bulb of Penis   The expanded portion of the third penile cylinder surrounding the urinary passage soon after it leaves the bladder.

Bulbospongiosus   One of a pair of muscles covering part of the base of the penis, under the bones of the pelvis.

Caffeine   A stimulant drug found in coffee, tea and cola drinks.

Chronic   Present for a long time.

Circumcision	An operation to remove the foreskin of the penis.
Clitoris	A tiny, very sexually sensitive structure at the top of a woman's genitals, which is the female equivalent of the penis.
Corona	The rear border of the head of the penis.
Corpus Cavernosum	The penile cylinder on each side of the penis concerned solely with erection. The 2 together are known as the corpora cavernosa.
Corpus Spongiosum	The penile cylinder surrounding the urinary passage.
Crus of Penis	The base of the corpus cavernosum of each side of the penis, located underneath, and attached to, the bones of the pelvis.
Desensitization	A psychological treatment for inappropriate anxiety (or inappropriate guilt, anger, and so on).
Detumescence	Subsidence of penile enlargement or erection.
Ejaculation	The expulsion of seminal fluid from the urinary passage to the exterior.
Endocrine Glands	Specialized body organs which produce hormones, which are then secreted into the blood stream.
Erectile	To do with getting or keeping an erection.
Erection	An enlargement of the penis beyond its resting size. This may or may not be to its maximum size (full or complete erection).
Fantasy	Imaginary scenes or series of thoughts; daydream.
Fetish	A personalized, specific object or situation, necessary for, or especially powerful in, producing sexual arousal.
Foreskin	The skin partially or completely covering the head of the penis, which is removed in the operation called circumcision.

Genitals	The external sexual organs involved in reproduction.
Glans Penis	The head of the penis or expanded end of the corpus spongiosum.
Hormone	A chemical produced by a gland in the body, which is necessary for the normal functioning of some other body organ or organs.
Implant	Inert material surgically imbedded in the body for a specific purpose.
Ischiocavernosus	One of a pair of muscles covering part of the base of the penis, under the bones of the pelvis.
Libido	Sexual interest or sexual drive.
Masturbation	Fondling one's own genitals to produce pleasurable feelings, and eventually orgasm.
Nerve	A specialized structure for conducting messages to and from the brain and spinal cord.
Nicotine	A toxic drug present in tobacco which can cause narrowing of blood vessels.
Orgasm	The sudden, intensely pleasurable feeling, which in men normally accompanies ejaculation, and which represents the height or climax of sexual arousal and enjoyment.
Pelvis	The basin-shaped ring of bones at the lower end of the trunk and the cavity encircled by them.
Placebo	A medicine which exerts a beneficial effect purely on a psychological basis. The benefit is not due to a genuine drug effect.
Potency	The ability to get an adequate erection when desired.
Premack Principle	A simple psychological procedure for making desired thoughts or behaviour occur more frequently.

Prepuce	Foreskin.
Prognosis	Outlook for cure or improvement.
Prosthesis (Penile)	A penile implant inserted into the erection chambers to produce an artificial erection.
Refractory Period	The time after an ejaculation or orgasm before a man can again achieve erection or ejaculation.
Scrotum	The bag of skin at the base of the penis containing the testicles.
Sedative	A drug which makes one calm and often drowsy.
Self-monitoring	Recording the occurrence of an undesired thought or behaviour, immediately after it occurs, resulting in a decrease in the future occurrence of the thought or behaviour recorded.
Sensuality	Awareness of, and pleasure in experiencing, one or more of the body's senses — touch, hearing, vision, taste and smell.
Spinal Cord	An extension of the brain down through the vertebral column (backbone).
Testicles	The two bird-egg sized structures hanging in the bag of skin lying at the base of the penis. They produce sperm cells and male hormone.
Testosterone	Male hormone.
Thought Stopping	A simple and effective psychological procedure for getting unwanted thoughts out of one's mind.
Tourniquet	Something tight placed around a part of the body to block the normal flow of blood.
Tranquillizer	A drug which calms without usually making one drowsy.
Tumescence	An enlargement of the penis due to extra blood in the erection chambers.

Tunica Albuginea   A thick pressure-resistant sheath surrounding each erection chamber.

Urethra   The tube through which urine passes from the bladder to the end of the penis.

Vagina   The female sexual passage, running from the external genitals to the womb.

Vein   A tube taking used blood away from a part of the body, back towards the heart.

Vertebral Column   The bones which sit one on top of each other to form the spine or backbone.

Vibrator   An electrical gadget, which when activated, produces rapid back and forward movement of either the whole device, or a portion of the device.

Index